Orthodontic Retainers and Removable Appliances

Principles of Design and Use

Orthodontic Retainers and Removable Appliances

Principles of Design and Use

Friedy Luther

BDS (Hons), FDS RCS Eng, D Orth RCS Eng, M Orth RCS Eng, MSc, PhD, F HEA
Consultant Orthodontist and Honorary Senior Clinical Lecturer
The Charles Clifford Dental Hospital
Sheffield Teaching Hospitals NHS Foundation Trust
Sheffield
UK

Zararna Nelson-Moon

MSc, PhD, BDS (Hons), MOrth RCS Eng, FDS Orth RCS Eng
Consultant Orthodontist
York Teaching Hospital NHS Foundation Trust
York
UK

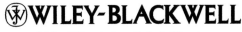

WILEY-BLACKWELL

A John Wiley & Sons, Ltd., Publication

This edition first published 2013
© 2013 by Friedy Luther and Zararna Nelson-Moon

Wiley-Blackwell is an imprint of John Wiley & Sons, formed by the merger of Wiley's global Scientific, Technical and Medical business with Blackwell Publishing.

Registered office: John Wiley & Sons, Ltd, The Atrium, Southern Gate, Chichester, West Sussex, PO19 8SQ, UK

Editorial offices: 9600 Garsington Road, Oxford, OX4 2DQ, UK
The Atrium, Southern Gate, Chichester, West Sussex, PO19 8SQ, UK
2121 State Avenue, Ames, Iowa 50014-8300, USA

For details of our global editorial offices, for customer services and for information about how to apply for permission to reuse the copyright material in this book please see our website at www.wiley.com/wiley-blackwell.

Library of Congress Cataloging-in-Publication Data

Luther, Friedy.

   Orthodontic retainers and removable appliances : principles of design and use / Friedy Luther, Zararna Nelson-Moon.
     p. ; cm.
   Includes bibliographical references and index.
   ISBN 978-1-4443-3008-3 (pbk. : alk. paper)
   I. Nelson-Moon, Zararna. II. Title.
   [DNLM: 1. Orthodontic Appliances, Removable. 2. Orthodontic Appliance Design. 3. Orthodontic Retainers. WU 426]

   617.6'43–dc23

2012022787

A catalogue record for this book is available from the British Library.

Wiley also publishes its books in a variety of electronic formats. Some content that appears in print may not be available in electronic books.

Cover images: left - courtesy of iStockphoto/© Dawn Poland; top right and bottom right - courtesy of the authors
Cover design by Meaden Creative

Set in 9.5/12 pt Palatino by Toppan Best-set Premedia Limited, Hong Kong

1   2013

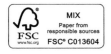

Contents

Preface

Why we need this book and who is it for?

This book aims to fill a gap in the literature that has existed for many years. Whilst it is a General Dental Council (GDC) requirement (quite rightly) to teach dental students orthodontic diagnosis and the principles of interceptive treatment (amongst other things), there seem to be no books that explain concisely, in practical terms (and in enough detail), what principles to apply when trying to design the appliances to enable this interceptive treatment to be undertaken. This book therefore sets out to address this.

Many books contain the principles but these are often obscured by excessive detail – or perhaps there is too much theory in the wrong place. Either way, things can get confusing. Alternatively, suggestions are made for 'standard appliances', but a one-size-fits-all approach is not always useful when it comes to working out when the 'standard appliance' is not appropriate. To reinforce this point, we also include a "Test yourself" chapter. Here, the reader can assess some patients for themselves and see whether or not a URA (upper removable appliance) would be appropriate or not.

In addition, in some cases, it may be necessary to refer a patient for specialist advice. For example, a patient may require initial, interceptive treatment but, in addition, may require referral for definitive treatment thereafter. It should be said that this would hopefully not be as a result of the interceptive treatment! Again, it is a GDC requirement that the dental graduate be competent at making appropriate referrals based on assessment. This is another aspect that this book gives advice on – what makes a good referral letter.

This book also includes a basic section on orthodontic retainers: current trends increasingly mean that patients wish to maintain their teeth as straight as possible following frequently lengthy, usually fixed, appliance treatment. Specialists performing orthodontic treatment must necessarily focus on the active treatment of the patients referred to them. Ultimately, such patients, if they wish to continue wearing retainers long term, need to be referred back to their own general dental practitioner (GDP) so they take over the responsibility of looking after their own patients and their patients' retainers. However, there is little, readily available information for the GDP to enable them to perform this duty. Therefore, this book aims to provide some basic guidance to address this.

In addition, there are a limited number of lower removable appliances (LRAs) which may have a use in certain, somewhat restricted, circumstances. These will be referred to at appropriate points in relevant chapters. For reasons of completeness, the book also includes chapters, specifically for the specialist trainee, on some other uses of removable appliances. These cover basic aspects of functional appliance design and the use of vacuum-formed active appliances (VFAAs; also known as aligners).

This book is thus aimed at dental undergraduates who have received basic training in orthodontic diagnosis; have a reasonable level of understanding; and are familiar with the basic terminology. However, we also intend it to be useful to postgraduate students of orthodontics; orthodontic therapists; qualified GDPs; orthodontic technicians, and postgraduates in paediatric dentistry – all of whom require a knowledge of interceptive orthodontic treatment.

Friedy Luther
Zararna Nelson–Moon

Acknowledgements

We have written this book in the hope that it will be useful to future generations of students of orthodontics. We have tried to achieve this by illustrating it as well as we possibly could. To this end, we have been reliant on the goodwill of fellow colleagues, clinicians and postgraduate students to help us obtain photographs (often at short notice), when we have not been able to obtain them ourselves. Jay Kindelan, Consultant Orthodontist at York (York Teaching Hospital NHS Foundation Trust) also helped us greatly by writing Chapter 11 for this book. We hope everyone will forgive us for badgering them.

However, above all we have been reliant on patients who have so kindly agreed to let us use their clinical photographs. We could not have produced this book without their willingness to help others.

We must also thank all the following colleagues and departments for all their help in supplying photographs or materials to be photographed. In no particular order, they are as follows.

At The Charles Clifford Dental Hospital, Sheffield Teaching Hospitals NHS Foundation Trust /School of Clinical Dentistry, University of Sheffield:

Fiona Dyer, Consultant Orthodontist;
Joanne Birdsall, Post-CCST Specialist Registrar;
Say Mei Lim, Staff Grade Orthodontist;
Peter Germain, SpR;
Rachel Norman and Jane Kilvington, Orthodontic Therapists.

At the Leeds Dental Institute/Leeds Teaching Hospitals NHS Trust/University of Leeds:
David Morris, Consultant Orthodontist;
Angus Robertson and the Team of Medical & Dental Illustration;
Michael Flynn and the Orthodontic Technicians;
Jacki Keasberry, Postgraduate Paediatric Dentistry student.

At St Luke's Hospital, Bradford/Bradford Teaching Hospitals NHS Foundation Trust:
Simon Littlewood, Consultant Orthodontist;
Carol Bentley, Orthodontic Therapist.

At York, York Teaching Hospital NHS Foundation Trust:
Sandra Hudson, Orthodontic Therapist;
Mike Pringle, Department of Medical Illustration.

Andrew DiBiase, Consultant Orthodontist, East Kent Hospitals University NHS Foundation Trust.

Thanks are also due to the following for their help:

Jancyn Gardiner for her timely legal advice;

Clearstep™ for permission to use some of the figures in Chapter 11 (as noted therein);

Oxford University Press (for permission to use Figure 2.1).

Finally, huge thanks must also go to our long-suffering partners and families who survived the ordeal as well as to our publishing team at Wiley-Blackwell who include: Sophia Joyce, Lucy Nash and Katrina Hulme-Cross.

Abbreviations

Throughout this text, the following abbreviations have been used:

EOT: extra-oral traction

FABP: flat anterior biteplane

FMPA: Frankfort–mandibular planes angle

GDC: General Dental Council

GDP: General Dental Practitioner

ICP: inter-cuspal position

IOTN: Index of Orthodontic Treatment Need

IPR: interproximal reduction

LLS: lower labial segment (usually taken to mean the lower incisors although some clinicians include the lower canines)

LRA: lower removable appliance

MOA: medium opening activator

PIL: patient information leaflet

RCP: retruded contact position

ss: stainless steel

ULS: upper labial segment (usually taken to mean the upper incisors although some clinicians include the upper canines)

URA: upper removable appliance (not to be confused with upper right deciduous central incisor, see below!)

VFAA: vacuum-formed active appliance

VFR: vacuum-formed retainer

In addition, readers should note that the commonly used abbreviation for a supernumerary tooth, $, is used.

Tooth notation: the alpha numeric tooth notation system will be used, e.g. upper right lateral incisor would be UR2. An upper right deciduous central incisor is noted as UR A.

Assumptions: What You Should Know and Understand Before You Use this Book

As a reader of this book, it is only fair that you know what you are getting as the remit is certainly not to teach orthodontics! It concentrates on discussing the practical aspects of only two, relatively discreet, but important aspects of orthodontics:

- **Interceptive treatment** deals with the developing, childhood dentition at a time when decisions can strongly influence long-term outcomes. Identifying and explaining the principles of interception are among the learning outcomes identified by the General Dental Council.
- **Retention** is an increasingly important part of orthodontic treatment for many patients. More and more, patients may wish to maintain (for as long as feasible) their treatment result following what may often have been lengthy and complex treatment. It is thus likely that general dental practitioners will need to take over the care and responsibility for their patients' retainer requirements. Incidentally, however, it should be noted

that whilst upper removable appliances (URAs) are appropriate for childhood interceptive treatment, they are not often useful for adults. In contrast, retainers may be worn by children or adults.

This book will also give pertinent advice on:

- **What makes a good referral letter** (again in line with the General Dental Council outcomes), e.g. when a patient requires referral to a specialist for definitive orthodontic treatment.
- **What is required when and the reasons for taking over the care and responsibility of a patient's retainer requirements**.

In addition, discussion of lower removable appliances (LRAs) is included where appropriate, as well as specific chapters for the specialist trainee.

The authors acknowledge that the practical advice given in this book will sometimes not exactly match that given by every clinician, but

Orthodontic Retainers and Removable Appliances: Principles of Design and Use, First Edition.
Friedy Luther and Zararna Nelson-Moon.
© 2013 Friedy Luther and Zararna Nelson-Moon. Published 2013 by Blackwell Publishing Ltd.

subtle differences in approach are evident between clinicians in all specialties. The approach adopted here is one that we have found works for us. Furthermore, as this is essentially a practical guide based on clinical experience, it is not written nor intended as a fully-referenced academic text.

So, this book assumes a basic level of orthodontic knowledge of the sort you would hopefully receive from an undergraduate dental training. This means that it does not explain terms such as overjet, overbite, the different skeletal, incisor or molar classifications, etc. – it will assume you know these already. It will also not explain how to undertake an orthodontic diagnosis, only pointing out aspects of diagnosis that are relevant to the particular problem under discussion.

Also this book will not explain how to undertake all orthodontic treatment. That is a specialist area. However, what this book will do is give guidance on situations where interceptive treatment could potentially be considered and how. Yet, this can never be comprehensive since no two patients are ever entirely identical. Many aspects of diagnosis can influence a decision as to whether a treatment is reasonable, possible or even feasible.

In addition, this book does not discuss issues of consent, risks of orthodontic treatment and balancing the risk/benefit ratio. These are all vital issues, but again we assume a level of knowledge that basic undergraduate dental training should cover.

Lastly and obviously, this book provides no direct practical experience whatsoever!

Upper Removable Appliances: Indications and Principles of Design

Upper removable appliances (URAs) are 're-movable braces' that fit on the upper arch only. In the past, URAs were used for many malocclusions, including severe Class II division 1 cases. However, this is no longer seen as appropriate because removable appliances can only achieve very simple movements, i.e. simple tipping of teeth, and the vast majority of malocclusions that warrant treatment require far more complex movements (using fixed appliances) to achieve an adequate outcome. Fixed appliances can also tip teeth, but in complete contrast to removable appliances, they can also achieve bodily movement (including rotations, intrusion and extrusion) as well as torque. Therefore, regarding active treatment, this book will mostly confine itself to interceptive treatment where the types of malocclusion to be intercepted are very limited; if tooth movement is required, it is confined to tipping movements. The exceptions are covered in Chapters 10 and 11.

> **Learning outcomes**
>
> After reading this chapter you should know:
>
> - The indications for the use of URAs
> - The importance of anchorage
> - The advantages and disadvantages of removable appliances
> - What the components of URAs are
> - What the components of URAs look like
> - The design principles and steps to consider when designing URAs
> - The importance of the timing of appointments

Prerequisites for orthodontic treatment

It must be understood that for *any* patient seeking *any form* of orthodontic treatment, dental health (including dietary control) *and* oral hygiene must be *excellent* prior to treatment.

Orthodontic Retainers and Removable Appliances: Principles of Design and Use, First Edition.
Friedy Luther and Zararna Nelson-Moon.
© 2013 Friedy Luther and Zararna Nelson-Moon. Published 2013 by Blackwell Publishing Ltd.

Therefore, before any referral is made, the referring dentist *must* ensure that their patient is dentally fit, i.e. no active caries, gingivitis or periodontal disease, and that they have a standard of oral hygiene that is excellent – this is the level required to support appliance therapy. A number of recent audits in the UK have indicated that 30% of patients have undiagnosed/untreated caries on referral to an orthodontist. This wastes a great deal of everyone's time as, obviously, the orthodontist cannot accept a patient for treatment if the patient is not dentally fit and/or has poor oral hygiene/diet control. This is because significant damage, e.g. caries, will be caused to the teeth and supporting structures by any appliance used under the wrong conditions. Damage will also occur far more quickly and severely than under normal conditons. Furthermore, restoration of teeth is more difficult once appliances are in place.

If, as the referring clinician, your patient cannot meet these conditions, but wants orthodontic treatment, you will need to explain to the patient/carers why referral is inappropriate and what the consequences of poor dental health are for their orthodontic treatment prospects. Treatment may be harder or more complicated if treatment has to be delayed until growth is (nearly) completed. Indeed, treatment may not be feasible unless dental health improves.

Oral hygiene that is less than optimal may lead to demineralisation of the enamel surface around or under any appliance, including the attachments of a fixed appliance. Such demineralisation can actually occur within a few weeks of an appliance being placed and, if severe, can lead to cavitation. The benefit of orthodontic treatment in providing a good occlusion and smile aesthetics is thus undone by the marking on the labial surfaces of the teeth in the case of fixed appliances (see Figure 5.20). However, around URAs damage may be hidden palatally from the patient and unwary clinician.

Moving teeth through bone in the presence of gingival inflammation and/or active periodontal disease will lead to very rapid destruction of the alveolar bone. Therefore, tooth movement should never be undertaken until the disease has been successfully treated; there is no bleeding from the gingival margins or the base of the periodontal pockets, and the patient has demonstrated that they are able to maintain the necessary level of oral hygiene.

It should be emphasised that before *any* appliance is fitted, a full orthodontic assessment (including appropriate radiographs) and diagnosis *must* have been performed. A problem list derived from the case assessment will then form the basis of a proper treatment plan. It is assumed that readers are able to undertake these tasks appropriately and the details of these steps are not covered here. To refresh your memory on any aspects of assessment, diagnosis or treatment planning, readers are referred to other textbooks.

Anchorage

Before discussing how to design URAs, we need to briefly remind ourselves about one very important aspect of orthodontic treatment – anchorage. Unless anchorage is given appropriate consideration, orthodontic treatment cannot only easily fail, but the original malocclusion can be made much worse.

What is anchorage?

Anchorage is most easily defined as the resistance to unwanted tooth movement. In other words, it is what stops the wrong teeth from moving. Newton's Third Law of Motion states that: 'To every action there is an equal and opposite reaction'.

In orthodontics, because of Newton's Third Law, we can all too easily find that unwanted tooth movement takes place. In order to minimise such movement, it is generally accepted that during URA treatment, only one or two teeth should be moved at a time. This means that the movement of a few teeth (or a tooth) is being pitted against the movement of many or the majority of teeth. This works because generally, the larger number of 'anchoring' teeth will have a larger root surface area than the smaller number of teeth to be moved (see Figure 2.1 for examples). Whilst the equal and opposite reaction will be 'experienced' by all the teeth in contact with the appliance, this force will be distributed according to root surface area. Thus, large rooted teeth will 'experience' a larger force than small rooted teeth, but if there are many teeth in contact, then each tooth will 'experience' relatively low force levels – levels that will not lead to significant tooth movement. Pitting a larger number of teeth against a smaller number of teeth actually being moved, thus provides increased anchorage. However, where for example a crossbite is to be corrected, it may be appropriate to pit one upper quadrant (e.g. URCDE6) against the opposite buccal quadrant using a screw as the active component. Turning the screw results in equal buccal movement of both sets of upper buccal teeth in a reciprocal movement since the root surface areas of both sets of teeth are roughly equivalent.

Causes of anchorage loss

In circumstances where anchorage is not controlled, it can be lost very easily.

Operator factors

* Incorrect diagnosis/treatment plan
* Over activation of springs
* Incorrect URA prescription, e.g. if wire dimensions are too thick, these apply too much force when activated
* Inappropriate spring design or inadequate/ ambiguous spring prescription on the laboratory card

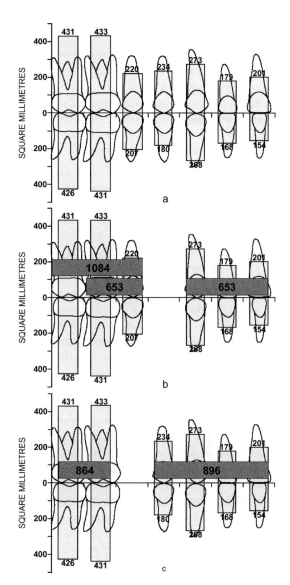

Figure 2.1 Anchorage. Larger teeth have larger root surface areas than smaller teeth. The groups of teeth that are pitted against each other will determine the anchorage balance. (Reproduced from Nelson-Moon ZL (2007) Craniofacial growth, cellular basis of tooth movement and anchorage. In: L Mitchell (ed) *An Introduction to Orthodontics*, p. 46, Figure 4.20, by permission of Oxford University Press.)

Patient factors

- Failure to wear appliance as instructed
- Distortion of spring(s) causing excessive force to be applied
- Appliance breakages, allowing uncontrolled tooth movement
- Failure to return for appliance checks, allowing uncontrolled tooth movement

Laboratory factors

- Failure to follow prescription
- Prescription unclear, leading to errors in manufacture

Results of anchorage loss

In the worst case scenario, treatment can make the original malocclusion far worse. For example, if one or more teeth is/are retracted distally along the arch using excessive forces, the other teeth, via the equal and opposite reaction, will move mesially. Especially if the force levels are sufficient to reach optimum levels (25–50 g), the 'anchorage' teeth will 'experience' forces leading to forward movement of all the anchorage teeth. This will appear as a visible and measurable increase in overjet. This increase in overjet will continue for as long as the excessive force is applied. In other words, it is possible for a patient who has a normal overjet to end up with an increased overjet as a *result of poor management or incompetence by the dentist. To put it bluntly, they could end up complaining of 'goofy teeth' – a problem caused by orthodontic treatment. Such problems can be very hard to correct. As can be seen from the lists above, operator causes of anchorage loss outnumber those caused by patients.*

Sources of anchorage

Anchorage is gained from all teeth in contact with the URA and from contact with the palate. Well-fitting appliances are thus crucial. Rarely, anchorage can be re-inforced using extra-oral sources, i.e. headgear. In addition, in a rela-tively new development that is beyond the remit of this book, anchorage may be gained in some circumstances using temporary anchorage devices (TADs; also known as mini-screws). These are now being used in conjunction with fixed appliances.

The remit of this book is limited. Therefore, readers are strongly advised to consult other textbooks for more detailed discussions of how anchorage can be gained and its management. However, anchorage will be discussed briefly in connection with the examples of appliance design given in Chapter 3.

Components of URAs

URAs always comprise an acrylic baseplate with various stainless-steel (ss) wire components. These wire components may have the following functions:

- **To retain (or 'clip') the appliance to the upper teeth.** All URAs will have these.
- **To move the teeth.** These active components are springs. Only active appliances will have these.
- **To prevent movement of some teeth.** These passive components simply hold the teeth still. These may be made of wire or acrylic and, whilst they will always be present on passive appliances, they may also be present on active appliances.

For some URAs, active components may use a screw rather than a spring to move teeth.

An example of a URA is shown in Figure 2.2. URAs are orthodontic appliances which, if active, *only tip* teeth or, if passive, *maintain* tooth position. That is *all* they do. This is in contrast to fixed appliances which, as we have already said, can perform all tooth movements (including tipping of teeth).

Passive URAs are of two types:

- **Space maintainers:** these aim to prevent the movement of teeth into a space where another tooth is to erupt.

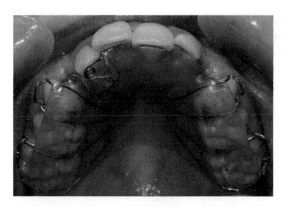

Figure 2.2 Example of an upper removable appliance (URA). This shows a Z-spring used for correcting incisor crossbites.

- **Retainers:** these aim to maintain teeth in their new positions following active tooth movement. They may also be used to hold open spaces that have been created during active treatment for restorative purposes, e.g. in patients with hypodontia. Retainers will be discussed separately in Chapters 7–9.

With the exception of some retainers (e.g. vacuum-formed retainers; see Chapters 7 and 8) and space-maintaining appliances, the components of all other URAs are:

- **Retentive components:** These are usually wire clasps, most commonly either Adams' clasps (for posterior or anterior teeth, hence their other name of 'universal' clasps) or Southend clasps (for one or two adjacent anterior teeth). Occasionally 'C'-clasps or some types of labial bow may be useful, but labial bows are mostly used in retaining appliances (retainers). Other types of retentive components also exist but are generally infrequently used. For instance, ball clasps can be used but generally only in quite specialist situations such as in the Twin Block functional appliance around the lower incisors (see Figure 10.3 and 10.4).

- **Acrylic baseplate:** This will be unmodified if the appliance is passive, but in active appliances may sometimes usefully include posterior capping or a biteplane.
- **Active components:** These are most frequently wire springs or occasionally screws; rarely a labial bow is used, but the indications (see Chapter 3) are very limited so it is better to dismiss bows for active tooth movement in most cases.

When tipping teeth with a URA, only light forces (25–50 g; 50 g maximum) per spring must be applied. The force applied by an activated spring can be measured with spring gauges as shown in Figure 2.3. URAs that incorporate springs as the active component rely on being activated by the clinician; this contrasts with screw appliances which have to be activated by the patient. The latter are therefore only used where a spring cannot easily be used, e.g. where several, adjacent teeth require tipping and several springs would make the appliance too complex to seat. Another situation is where retention is at a premium. A disadvantage of screws is that they tend to apply a larger, less controlled force than a spring.

What are the indications for the use of URAs?

Remember that active URAs can only tip teeth. The indications can thus be summarised as in Table 2.1, assuming that tipping is the appropriate movement where active tooth movement is required.

Advantages and disadvantages of removable appliances

Advantages

- **Anchorage efficient:** unlike fixed appliances, they gain anchorage from palatal contact.

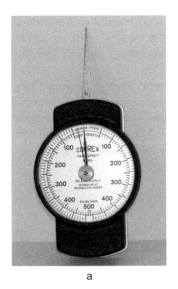
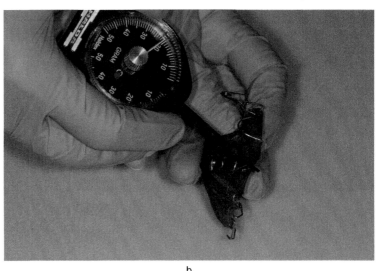

a   b

Figure 2.3 Examples of spring gauges. Both (a) extra-oral and (b) intra-oral versions exist. The intra-oral gauge is being used to measure the force applied by an activated palatal finger spring.

Table 2.1 Indications for the use of active and passive URAs.

Active	Passive
Expansion by tipping	Space maintainers
Tipping teeth mesially/ distally along the arch	Retainers
Tipping teeth labially/ buccally	
Reduction of overbite	
Reduction of overjet	

- **Less chairside time:** laboratory construction should mean that fitting is simple and quick with only minimal adjustments required.
- **Efficient overbite reduction:** all lower posterior teeth are free to over-erupt – providing the appliance is worn as instructed.
- **Can move blocks of teeth:** this is possible using a screw plate.

- **Easier to maintain good oral hygiene** (at least in theory though this does not always translate into reality): the appliance must and can be removed for cleaning.
- **Useful in mixed dentition:** URAs can be trimmed and retained to accommodate or fit around/avoid exfoliating deciduous teeth.

Disadvantages

- **Rely on patient co-operation:** if the patient does not wear the URA as instructed, then treatment cannot progress satisfactorily.
- **Oral hygiene:** likewise, oral hygiene and dental health can easily be compromised if the patient is not rigorous in following cleaning advice. This can occur despite the fact that the appliance is removable. Equally, the clinician is responsible for advising the patient when and where oral hygiene is sub-optimal.
- **Can only tip teeth:** teeth requiring any movement other than tipping require fixed appliances.

- **Affect speech:** this is only a temporary problem if the URA is worn properly.
- **Require laboratory production:** this involves time and expense but should at least make the fit appointment easy.

Design

Laboratory prescription

An essential part of designing any removable appliance is to be able to prescribe the design appropriately on the laboratory card. In all cases, rather in the same way partial dentures are prescribed, all components need to be first drawn out on the laboratory card and then given a written description.

The diagrammatic prescription should show:

- The design of the wire components to be used
- The baseplate plus any baseplate modifications that may be needed
- The placement of any screws if used and where the acrylic should be split
- Which tooth/teeth it applies to.

The written description should:

- Name the components (be they wire-work or baseplate modification)

- Describe the diameter of the ss wire to be used for each component
- Describe the layout of any baseplate modifications required, e.g. ½ occlusal coverage posterior capping UR and UL DE6
- Indicate which tooth or teeth it applies to, whether it is a wire component or baseplate modification
- Give any other useful or helpful comments, e.g. 'If enough undercut, please place Adams' clasp on URD; otherwise use double clasp on URE6'.

In this way the technician is given precise detail of the exact layout, appearance and construction of the appliance – both in diagrammatic form and in words. The two complementary sets of instruction should therefore back each other up. If they do not, then the technician has immediate grounds for querying the prescription with the clinician to clarify any ambiguities.

How the components are drawn on the laboratory cards and how the written instructions should be prescribed are shown in Figures 2.4, 2.5, 2.6, 2.7, 2.8, 2.9, 2.10 and 2.11, and in Chapter 3.

This chapter will now take a step-by-step approach to work through how any URA

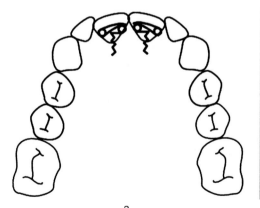
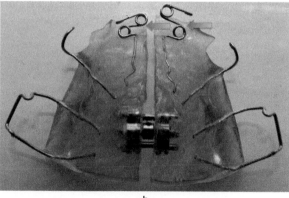

a   b

Figure 2.4 Z-springs drawn on the laboratory card (a) and an example of Z-springs (b; arrowed) on this appliance (which also shows C-clasps and Adams' clasps).

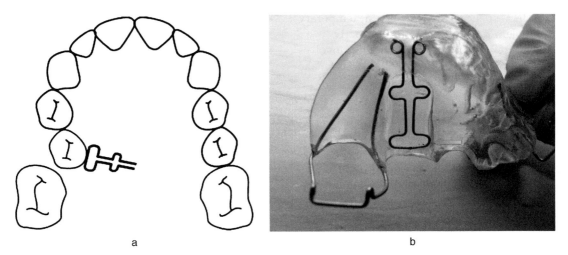

a   b

Figure 2.5 T-springs drawn on the laboratory card (a) and an example of a T-spring (b; arrowed) on this appliance (which also shows an Adams' clasp).

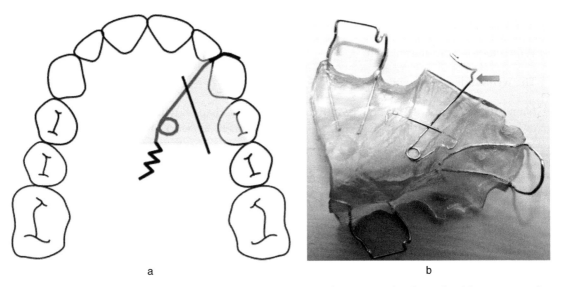

a   b

Figure 2.6 Palatal finger springs drawn on the laboratory card (a). Example of a palatal finger spring (b; arrowed) (which also shows the spring's box and guard wire, Adams' clasps and a modified Southend clasp, which engages one tooth only).

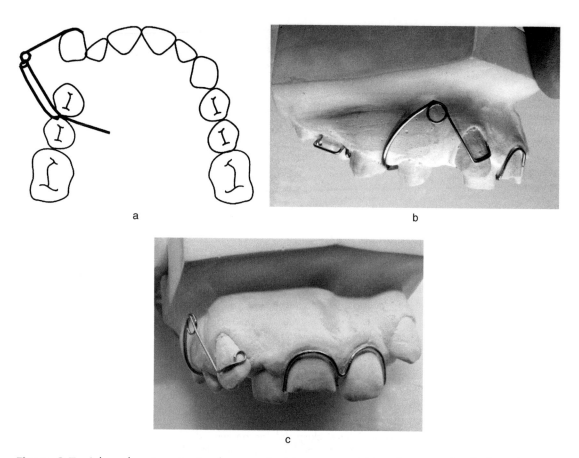

Figure 2.7   A buccal canine retractor drawn on the laboratory card (a) and an example of a buccal canine retractor (b and c) (which also show a Southend clasp on the central incisors and an Adams' clasp).

should be designed. A well-known acronym is ARAB: **A**ctive, **R**etention, **A**nchorage and **B**aseplate. It provides a simple checklist of the steps we need to consider.

A: Active components

It is assumed you have decided which tooth/ teeth to move, so the next step is to consider how best to perform the active tooth movement(s), i.e. what active component(s) to use.

What are the choices?

Nowadays, the only realistic choices are between springs and screws. Springs should be considered as the first choice because they are:

- Activated only by the operator (hence, unlike screw appliances, they do not rely on the co-operation of the patient)
- Less bulky than screws
- Cheaper than screws.

Conversely, if tipping several teeth at the same time and in the same direction, a screw appliance is usually preferable because appliances with multiple springs are complex and difficult for the patient to fit.

- Screws have one unique advantage in one situation. This is where retention is at a premium and it is required to retain the appliance *using the teeth to be moved*. In these

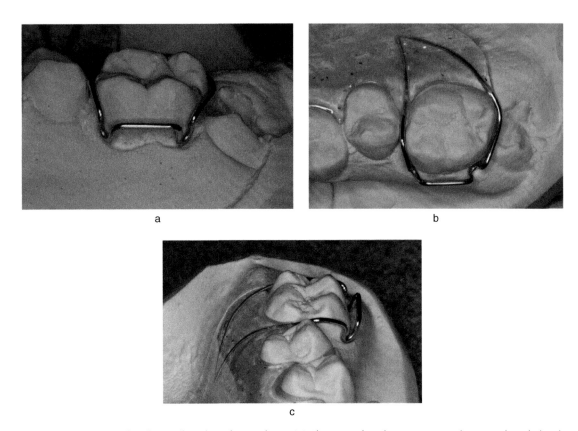

a

b

c

Figure 2.8   Example of a well-made Adams' clasp. (a) The arrowheads must enage the mesial and distal buccal undercuts. (b) The bridge does not project too far away from or too closely to the buccal surface of the molar. (c) The fly-overs lie right down in the embarsures. These features enable good retention whilst maximising comfort and ease of use both for patient and clinician. See Figure 2.13 for the laboratory card representation of Adams' clasps.

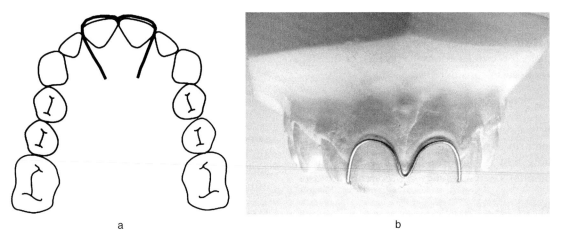

a

b

Figure 2.9   A Southend clasp drawn on the laboratory card (a) and its clinical appearance (b).

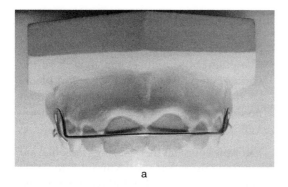

a

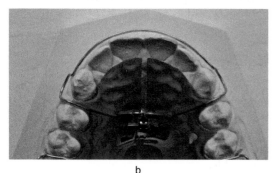

b

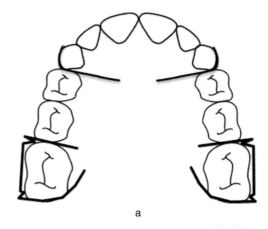

a

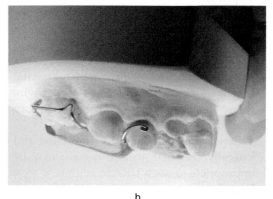

b

Figure 2.11 A C-clasp drawn on the laboratory card (a) and an example of a C-clasp (b) (see also Figure 2.4).

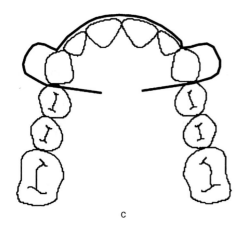

c

Figure 2.10 Example of a labial bow with U-loops (a) from the front and (b) occlusally. (c) Drawn on a laboratory card.

circumstances, a screw appliance is the only option if anything at all is to be used.
- However, screws do rely entirely on patient understanding and co-operation; they are also bulky and expensive.

In the past, elastics were used – even between upper and lower removable appliances, with predictably hopeless results as the lower removable appliance was dislodged and sprang off the teeth! They were also used within the arch to reduce an overjet, but could slip unnoticed under the gingivae or provide an unpleasant-looking 'flattened off' appearance across the front of the arch. Nowadays, however, elastics are much more usefully combined with URAs when extruding a surgically exposed tooth or partially erupted tooth.

Various bows (such as Robert's retractors) have been used to reduce overjets, but the need to achieve high quality results should make them virtually redundant in contemporary ortho-dontics. This is because overjets need to be reduced by careful tooth movement with indi-vidual bodily control, so that over-retroclination can be avoided. This means that fixed appliances are almost always by far the more appropriate choice.

Recommendations

- **For tipping anterior teeth over the bite,** we recommend Z-springs (they fit the palatal contour of the anterior teeth better than T-springs).
- **For pushing buccal teeth over the bite,** we recommend T-springs (they fit the palatal contour better than Z-springs).
- **For moving teeth mesially or distally along the line of the arch,** we recommend palatal finger springs with a box and guard wire (these must be specified on the laboratory prescription and are described below).
- **Where a canine is mesially angulated and buccally crowded,** in rare cases it may be appropriate to use a URA to align it. If so, a buccal canine retractor should be used. However, control may not be ideal and often a fixed appliance would deliver a better result. A palatal finger spring should not be used as this will cause the tooth to rotate due to its inability to contact the tooth appropri-ately, as there would have to be a long span of unsupported, thin wire.

Box and guard wire

It is vital that any spring is made as stable as pos-sible, i.e. that it presses on the tooth in such a way that it only applies force in the direction planned/anticipated. Obviously, there are limits to this, but it is essential that palatal finger springs lie in a V-shaped channel (the box) cut out of the acrylic. In addition, a guard wire is positioned over the free length of the wire before it emerges from the baseplate. These two design features provide the following advantages:

- Protect the spring from distortion
- Allow free, unobstructed movement (if the box is made properly)
- The guard wire reduces the chances of the spring being distorted in the vertical plane, i.e. it helps maintain its appropriate position on the contact point of the relevant tooth.

Examples of what these springs look like are shown in Figures 2.4, 2.5, 2.6 and 2.7, together with how the springs should be drawn on the laboratory card.

R: Retention

Now consider how the appliance is to stay in. The golden rule is that there must *always* (there are *no* exceptions) be anterior *and* posterior retention. This does not mean clasps *must* only be on U1s – it just means *as far forward (anteriorly)* as possible.

What types of retentive components are there?

Retention is almost always via Adams' clasps (for posterior or anterior teeth; Figure 2.8), Southend clasps (usually for two adjacent ante-rior teeth, but can be used on a single, anterior tooth; Figure 2.9) or occasionally a labial bow (for anterior teeth; Figure 2.10). C-clasps may also be a possibility (see Figures 2.4b and 2.11).

Posterior retention is almost always very easy to locate as, invariably, Adams' clasps can and should be placed on both U6s. Where anterior retention can be placed will be deter-mined by:

- The type of teeth present (and to an extent their position – it may not be possible to clasp rotated teeth)
- Their condition
- The amount of space needed to undertake the active tooth movement.

How should the retentive components be positioned?

We need to think about two key points:

- **The overall layout of the distribution**, e.g. what shape the distribution should form, such as a rectangle or triangle (Figures 2.12 and 2.13).
- **Whether there is space and where the space is to move the teeth we want to move.** For example, consider the situation where a lateral incisor is to be pushed over the bite. If there is only just enough space for the tooth to move between U1 and U3 or UC, then a clasp must not be put on either of the teeth adjacent to U2. This is because the fly-overs (the wire from the clasps that passes between the contact points) will encroach on the space needed for U2 to move forward and this will prevent U2 from moving.

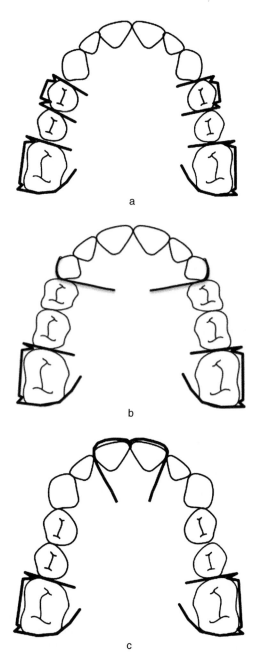

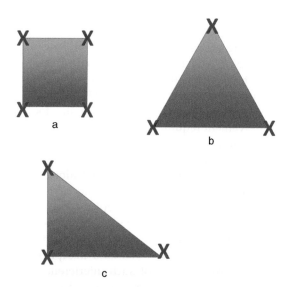

Figure 2.12 Retention can be placed so the clasps take up roughly the following shapes around the arch: rectangular/square (a) or triangular configuration (b and c).

Figure 2.13 Examples of the retention layouts of square/rectangular and triangular configuration drawn on a laboratory card (a–c, respectively).

Overall layout of retention distribution

Remember: the golden rule is that there must *always* (there are *no* exceptions) be anterior *and* posterior retention. Placement of the anterior retention on the upper central incisors is often ideal as it maximally reduces the chance of the appliance rocking.

This means that retention can be placed so the clasps take up roughly any of the following shapes:

* Rectangular
* Square
* Triangular configuration. In this case the base of the triangle should always be between UR6 and UL6 or, in unusual circumstances, between an U6 on one side and an U7 on the other.

For example, depending on the circumstances, Adams' clasps (or other types of retentive clasp) could be placed on both U6s and both U4s or UDs (rectangular configuration); both U6s and both U3s or UCs (a squarer configuration); or both U6s and UR12 (a variety of the triangular configuration). Other possibilities are essentially variations on this theme. Examples of possible retention layouts are shown diagrammatically in Figure 2.12 and as they could appear on a laboratory card in Figure 2.13.

A: Anchorage

Now the second 'A', which stands for anchorage. This has been discussed above and you should revise this section. Remember that Newton's Third Law of Motion states that 'To every action there is an equal and opposite reaction' and that anchorage can be defined as the resistance to unwanted tooth movement. Anchorage should be planned as part of the overall treatment plan. A more detailed description of anchorage is beyond the scope of this book, although some brief details are given for the specific URA designs in Chapter 3.

B: Baseplate

Finally, we need to consider the baseplate. Baseplates are either plain and unmodified or they are modified using posterior capping or a flat anterior biteplane.

Why might the baseplate need modifying?

Consider whether or not the tooth movements you want to undertake can actually occur without discluding the upper and lower teeth.

* **If they can,** then there is no need to modify the baseplate by way of variation in thickness.
* **If they cannot,** think about what is needed long term. There are two things to consider:
  * If in the long-run it would be better if the overbite is as good as now or even a little deeper, then opt for posterior capping.
  * If in the long-run it would be better (or acceptable) that the overbite is less than now, then opt for an anterior biteplane.

As rough rules of thumb only, it is more likely that:

* **Where a crossbite is to be corrected,** posterior capping will be needed. Special attention to trimming is needed when a single-tooth buccal crossbite is to be corrected (e.g. an U5), so as to avoid interfering with the tooth movement required whilst at the same time discluding the teeth to allow the relevant tooth to move.
* **Where a tooth is to be moved along the arch,** i.e. mesially or distally, either no modification or a thin anterior biteplane is needed. To confirm this, check to see whether occlusal interferences will prevent the requisite movement if only a standard baseplate is fitted. An example of such interferences is where a lateral incisor has drifted into the space of an unerupted U1 and needs to be tipped back, e.g. due to late diagnosis of a supernumerary.

What does posterior capping do?

Acrylic posterior capping covers the occusal surfaces of all the relevant upper buccal teeth either entirely or half way across the occlusal surface (see Figure 2.14a and b). This has two implications:

- **The anterior teeth are discluded.** This is necessary when an anterior crossbite is to be corrected. Failure to disclude will mean no movement of an anterior tooth or, worse still, movement of an anterior tooth into the lingual surface of a lower tooth.
- **The lower buccal teeth will occlude onto the capping**, leaving the lower labial segment (LLS), i.e. lower incisors, free to erupt. This means that the overbite could potentially increase due to LLS eruption (Figure 2.15a and b).

In the case of crossbite correction, posterior capping is usually welcome since stable crossbite correction requires a reasonable depth of overbite in the first place. This is due to the physical overlap of the lower incisors by the uppers. If no or only minimal overbite is present, then there is little or no likelihood of stability since overbite will inevitably reduce as the upper incisors are pushed forward. This is due to the arc on which they move and also some intrusion of the tooth due to the position of the spring on the cingulum plateau.

The main exception is likely to be where the overbite is already deep or is increased. In this situation, whilst posterior capping will still disclude the teeth, the side effect is that the overbite will be *even deeper* following correction of the crossbite. Careful consideration is therefore needed as to whether posterior capping is appropriate in these circumstances.

What does an anterior biteplane do?

An acrylic anterior biteplane is usually known as a 'flat anterior biteplane' (FABP) as it is simply a flat layer of acrylic that is built up behind the upper anterior teeth (Figures 2.16a and b, and 2.17). It is important to note that the overjet *must* be noted on the laboratory

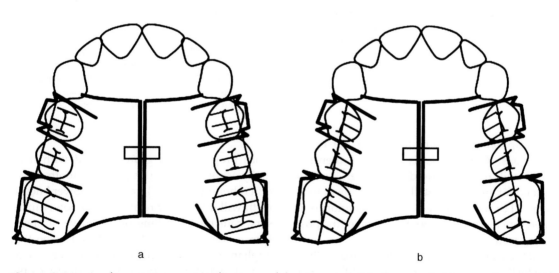

a b

Figure 2.14 Acrylic posterior capping drawn on a laboratory card. It is drawn so that it covers the occusal surfaces of all the relevant upper buccal teeth ('full occlusal coverage', a) or half way across the occlusal surface ('½ occlusal covarage', b). Usually it is preferable to request ½ occlusal covarage as this helps with oral hygiene and also allows easier adjustment of the clasps, etc. for the operator.

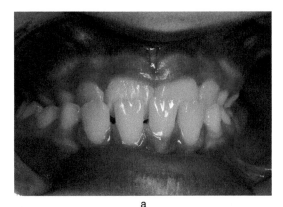

a

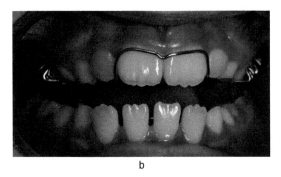

b

Figure 2.15 The effects of posterior capping on the occlusion. (a) An incisor crossbite prior to fitting a URA with posterior capping. (b) The patient is now fully discluded due to the URA carrying posterior capping. This allows forward movement of the upper incisors without hindrance from the lower incisors. It also allows for possible eruption of the lower incisors, which may be helpful in maintaining crossbite correction once the appliance is discarded.

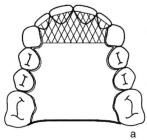

OJ = 8 mm
Please extend FABP
11 mm posteriorly
Depth = 2/3 height upper
central incisors

a

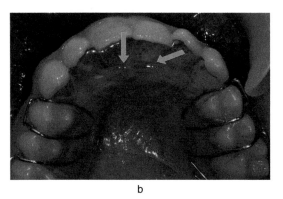

b

Figure 2.16 A flat anterior biteplane drawn on a laboratory card (a) and a biteplane in use in the mouth (b; note the wear facets caused by the lower incisors, arrowed). It is essential that the overjet (OJ) is noted on the laboratory prescription (as shown) to ensure the FABP functions correctly. If the OJ is *not* noted, then the FABP will not be made deep enough, i.e. it will not extend far enough palatally, the lower incisors (LLS) will occlude behind/posterior to it and there will be no disclusion of the posterior teeth. The height of the biteplane must also be specified to ensure it is sufficiently high to allow posterior disclusion of the buccal teeth by approximately 2–3 mm.

prescription (as shown) to ensure the FABP functions. If the overjet is *not* noted, then the FABP will not be made deep enough, i.e. not extend far enough palatally, and the lower incisors (LLS) will occlude behind/posterior to it; therefore there will be no disclusion of the posterior teeth.

If the patient's overjet *is* noted properly, then the FABP can be made properly and the lower incisors will occlude onto the FABP, leaving the lower posterior teeth free of occlusion and hence able to erupt (Figure 2.17). If an FABP is

worn properly by a growing child with normally erupting teeth, this posterior tooth eruption is bound to take place and the lower buccal teeth will over-erupt relative to the lower incisors, causing a levelling of the curve of Spee. Hence, the overbite will be reduced when the appliance is discontinued. Whether or not it remains reduced is dependent on various factors. However, providing the lower incisors occlude onto the palatal surface of the upper incisors and the inter-incisal angle is within normal

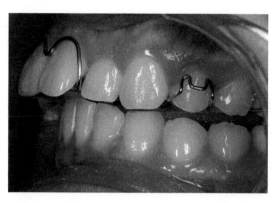

Figure 2.17 A flat anterior biteplane being used clinically. Note that if requested and constructed appropriately, the lower incisors bite onto the biteplane, resulting in the posterior buccal teeth being free of occlusion by about 2–3 mm. They are thus 'free to erupt' and this enables flattening of the occlusal plane. Due to wear, the biteplane may need to be built up from time to time in order to allow further overbite reduction if needed.

limits, then permanent overbite reduction is at least likely.

Therefore, an FABP should only be used where long-term reduction in the overbite will be acceptable (i.e. does no harm).

Now, to finish designing our appliance, we need to clear up a few other points.

What wire should be prescribed?

All wires in URAs are made of stainless steel and the dimensions given on the laboratory design sheets refer to wire diameters. The diameter of wire prescribed affects the force applied according to the equation:

$$\text{Force (F)} \propto dr^4 / l^3$$

where d = deflection, r = radius of wire and l = length.

It can be seen that as the radius/diameter of the wire increases, the force applied for the same length of wire and for the same deflection (activation) will be far greater than for the standard radius. It should therefore be apparent how important providing the correct prescription is.

Retentive components

Adams' clasps are made of 0.7 mm ss; the only exception is for small teeth (e.g. a deciduous molar) when it should be 0.6 mm ss.

Active/spring components

Any spring that is moving only one tooth is made of ss wire of diameter 0.5 mm.

Any spring that is moving two teeth, e.g. two adjacent upper incisors simultaneously or a single very large tooth (e.g. a molar), should be made of ss wire of diameter 0.6 mm or even 0.7 mm ss.

In the next chapter, we will look at examples where URAs could be used to good effect. In Chapter 6 you will have a chance to test yourself and see how well you have grasped the principles of URA design.

Cases Suitable for Treatment with Removable Appliances

3

Historically in the UK, removable appliances were used to treat a wide range of malocclusions, often to an acceptable standard when used by an experienced and skilled operator. However, it is now recognised that fixed appliances are able to achieve far superior results when used by operators trained in their use, and these have superseded removable appliances in many cases.

That said, the use of removable appliances is an extremely effective and efficient method of treatment in specific situations. These situations mostly relate to mixed dentition/interceptive orthodontics. They are very seldom indicated for definitive treatment of a malocclusion.

The majority of examples in this chapter will relate to upper removable appliances (URAs), although two examples of the use of a lower removable appliance (LRA) will be included. LRAs are less well tolerated by the patient than URAs because they encroach on tongue space. Also, it is more difficult to achieve good retention of a LRA because the undercuts on the lower molars are on the lingual side of the teeth, rather than the buccal side as for the upper molars. Often, the arrowheads of Adams' clasps on lower molars and premolars do not have any undercuts into which to engage, significantly reducing the retentive ability of the clasps.

> **Learning outcomes**
>
> After reading this chapter you should:
>
> - Have knowledge of the types of malocclusion that may be successfully treated with removable appliances
> - Be able to design removable appliances for treatment of a number of specific malocclusions
> - Understand the rationale behind specific design features
> - Be able to write out a laboratory prescription for your technician

Orthodontic Retainers and Removable Appliances: Principles of Design and Use, First Edition.
Friedy Luther and Zararna Nelson-Moon.
© 2013 Friedy Luther and Zararna Nelson-Moon. Published 2013 by Blackwell Publishing Ltd.

Expansion

In general terms, transverse expansion of the upper arch may be undertaken to correct unilateral or bilateral posterior crossbites in the following circumstances:

- There is a lateral displacement of the mandible on closure.
- Space is required in the upper arch to relieve crowding or aid in overjet reduction.
- The teeth that are to be moved are tipped palatally, i.e. bodily movement is not needed.

It is not always necessary to correct a posterior crossbite under other circumstances. However, when it is decided that crossbite correction is needed, it is always essential to assess:

- How much expansion is required to correct a crossbite
- Whether these tooth movements may be achieved
- The stability of the result.

Relapse of a posterior crossbite correction may leave the patient with a cusp-to-cusp relationship of the buccal teeth and, hence, induce a lateral mandibular displacement on closure. This is the reason why URAs should only be used to correct posterior crossbites in specific situations.

Design 1: Midline expansion screw (Figure 3.1)

Indications

- Bilateral narrowing of the maxillary arch in which the teeth are tipped palatally

This is often associated with a cusp-to-cusp buccal segment transverse relationship in the retruded contact position (RCP), leading to a lateral mandibular displacement into the intercuspal position (ICP) on closure. This could occur as a result of a digit-sucking habit.

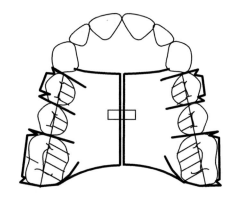

Please construct a URA to expand the upper arch:

1. Midline expansion screw
2. Adams' clasps UR6, UL6 – 0.7 mm hard ss wire
3. Adams' clasps URD, ULD – 0.6 mm hard ss wire
4. ½ occlusal coverage posterior capping
5. Midline split in baseplate as indicated
6. Baseplate saddled as indicated

Figure 3.1 Laboratory prescription for a URA that will provide symmetrical expansion of the upper arch.

- When a mandibular displacement on closure is present, clinically the patient presents with a unilateral posterior cross-bite on the side to which the mandible is displacing and a lower centre-line shift to the same side.
- The aim of the treatment is to expand the upper arch so that the cusp-to-cusp relationship is removed and the mandibular displacement eliminated.
- The points above illustrate why it is not always appropriate to correct a unilateral crossbite with 'unilateral' or asymmetric expansion (see Design 2 below and Figure 3.2). Therefore, it is essential that the presence of any mandibular displacement is detected prior to the design of the appliance.

Rationale: Correcting a posterior crossbite may help relieve crowding. Also, correcting a posterior

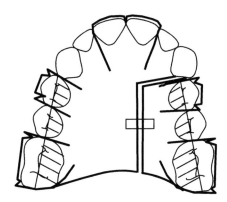

Please construct a URA to expand the upper arch:

1. Expansion screw positioned as shown to move ULDE6 directly buccally

2. Adams' clasps UR6, UL6 – 0.7 mm hard ss wire

3. Adams' clasps URD, ULD – 0.6 mm hard ss wire

4. Southend clasp UR1, UL1 – 0.7 mm hard ss wire

5. ½ occlusal coverage posterior capping

6. Split in baseplate as indicated

Figure 3.2 Laboratory prescription for a URA that will provide asymmetrical expansion of the upper arch.

crossbite that has been caused by a mandibular displacement during the early mixed dentition hopefully will enable subsequent permanent teeth to erupt into the RCP, so ensuring that any future orthodontic treatment is more straightforward. Other suggested adverse consequences of a lateral mandibular displacement on closure include tooth wear and the possibility of a young patient's mandible and hence dentition growing in an asymmetric pattern.

Contra-indications

* The buccal teeth are already buccally tipped (flared)

Rationale:

* The action of the removable appliance is to tip the teeth buccally to correct the transverse discrepancy. If the teeth are already tipped buccally, then only a limited amount of tooth movement is possible.
* As the teeth are tipped buccally, it causes the palatal cusp to 'drop down' and this has the effect of propping the bite open. This should be avoided especially in patients who have increased vertical dimensions.
* If the teeth are already buccally tipped, the presence of a posterior crossbite indicates a significant skeletal discrepancy between the maxilla and the mandible in the transverse dimension, and a removable appliance is not capable of correcting significant skeletal discrepancies.
* A bilateral posterior crossbite also indicates a significant transverse skeletal discrepancy and removable appliances should not be used for expansion in such cases.

Design features (Figure 3.1)

Active: Midline expansion screw.

Retention: Adams' clasps on upper first permanent molars (0.7 mm hard ss wire) and upper first premolars (0.7 mm wire) or upper first primary molars (0.6 mm wire).

Anchorage: Reciprocal: both sides of the arch will move by the same amount in a buccal direction.

Baseplate:
Midline split to allow expansion.
½ occlusal coverage posterior capping to disengage occlusion and allow free movement of upper teeth.

* Because of occlusal interferences between the maxillary and mandibular teeth, failure to disclude the teeth in a well-inter-digitated occlusion often results in concomitant

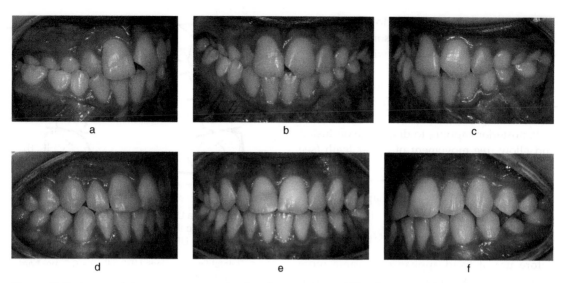

Figure 3.3 Intra-oral views, pre-treatment (a–c) and post-treatment (d-f), of a patient who underwent expansion of the upper arch with a URA in order to correct the crossbite of URCDE6. A Z-spring was used to correct the crossbite of UR2. Note the improvement in lower centre-line discrepancy. Also note that the patient requires no further orthodontic intervention as the permanent teeth have now erupted into a very acceptable position.

expansion of the lower arch, with no correction of the transverse discrepancy between the two

- Posterior capping will encourage the incisors to erupt and so will increase the overbite. If the overbite is already increased and a further increase is contra-indicated, then a flat anterior biteplane (FABP) may be included instead of posterior capping

Fitting and activation: See Chapter 4.

Design 2: Asymmetric expansion screw (Figure 3.2)

Indications

- Expansion of the upper arch where it is apparent that the narrowing of the maxillary arch is unilateral and there is a displacement of the mandible on closure

Once again, expansion may help relieve crowding and will hopefully enable subsequent permanent teeth to erupt into the RCP, so ensuring that any future orthodontic treatment is more straightforward (Figure 3.3).

Contra-indications

As above.

Design features (see Figure 3.2)

Active: Expansion screw, offset toward the side that requires expansion.

Retention: Adams' clasps on upper first permanent molars (0.7 mm hard ss wire) and upper first premolars (0.7 mm hard ss wire) or upper first primary molars (0.6 mm hard ss wire).

Southend clasp on upper central incisors (0.7 mm hard ss wire).

Anchorage: Because more teeth are included in the anchor unit, i.e. the teeth that do not need to be moved, there will be more expansion of the smaller unit – the teeth that do need moving. However, it is inevitable that some expansion of the teeth in the anchor unit will occur.

Baseplate: Split in baseplate to separate the teeth that need to be moved from the anchor unit.

½ posterior capping to disengage occlusion and allow free movement of upper teeth (see above).

Fitting and activation: See Chapter 4.

Moving teeth around the arch

Before use of fixed appliances became more common, removable appliances were often used to retract canines into the space created by the extraction of the first premolars as part of the treatment of Class II division 1 malocclusions. These days, because fixed appliances give such superior results, removable appliances are more commonly used simply to re-open space for the eruption of teeth by moving adjacent teeth around the arch, often in the mixed dentition.

Teeth can be moved mesially or, more commonly, distally, depending on requirements, but often space will need to be created first by the extraction of teeth, e.g. primary canine teeth.

Design 1: Use of palatal finger springs (Figure 3.4)

Indications

* Re-creation/redistribution of space, e.g. following loss of space for the eruption of a central incisor whose eruption has been impeded by a supernumerary tooth, and where the contra-lateral central incisor and the lateral incisors have tipped mesially into the unerupted central incisor space

  Rationale: An unerupted tooth will only erupt if there is enough room for it to do so and once two-thirds to three-quarters of its

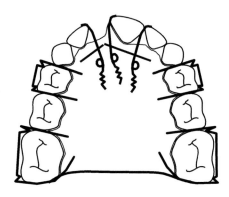

Please construct a URA to retract (distalise) the upper lateral incisors and the upper left central incisor to re-open space for UR1:

1. Palatal finger springs UR2, UL12 – 0.5 mm hard ss wire with box and guard wire

2. Adams' clasps UR6, UL6 – 0.7 mm hard ss wire

3. Adams' clasps URD, ULD – 0.6 mm hard ss wire

4. Baseplate saddled as indicated

Figure 3.4 Laboratory prescription for a URA to retract UR2, UL1 and UL2 to recreate space to allow the eruption of UR1.

root is formed. The teeth adjacent to a space will always tip into it. Therefore, the erupted incisors in this type of case are usually mesially tipped. The distal tipping caused by the springs serves to upright the teeth again, so achieving a more normal angulation at the same time as recreating the space. In this situation, it is often necessary to extract the primary canine teeth bilaterally to provide space into which to move the lateral incisor teeth.

* Retraction (distal movement) of canines that are in the line of the arch

  This should only be undertaken in rare and very specific cases where there is a small amount of space distal to the permanent canine teeth once they have erupted (up to 2–3 mm) and the canines are mesially tipped.

Rationale: This situation may be seen in cases where the upper permanent lateral incisors are microdont and the canines have tipped forward into the space. Tipping them distally again will create space distal to the upper laterals to allow composite build-ups on these teeth and so improve aesthetics.

Contra-indications

- Retraction of canines following the extraction of first premolar teeth
  Rationale: In general, canines should not be retracted into the space created by the extraction of the first premolar teeth using a URA, as this causes the crown of the canine to become distally angulated. This is unaesthetic and the root apex is left in its original position, leading to relapse. These cases should be treated using fixed appliances, which can control the crown angulation and root position.
- Retraction of teeth that are upright or distally angulated prior to treatment
  Rationale: The same principles apply as for retracting canines following extraction of premolar teeth.
- Retraction of buccally displaced canines
  Rationale: Palatal finger springs will push the tooth further from the line of the arch.

Design features of a URA to recreate space for the unerupted UR1 (see Figure 3.4)

Active: Palatal finger springs on the erupted central incisor and lateral incisors (0.5 mm wire) with box and guard wire (see Chapter 2).

Retention: Adams' clasps on the upper first permanent molars (0.7 mm hard ss wire) and upper first premolars (0.7 mm hard ss wire) or upper first primary molars (0.6 mm hard ss wire).

Anchorage: Care needs to be taken with the anchorage in this case. The reaction to the force applied to the incisor teeth to move them distally will be movement of the anchor teeth and the appliance mesially. Activating all three finger springs simultaneously will run the risk of losing anchorage and so disrupting the buccal segment relationship (it will become more Class II, i.e. move forward) and increasing the overjet.

Baseplate: The acrylic on the fit surface, around the finger springs, should be boxed out to ensure uninhibited activation of the springs (see Chapter 2). The collets distal to the incisors should be removed to allow distal movement of these teeth. If the overbite is increased, then an FABP may be included as appropriate.

Fitting and activation: See Chapter 4.

Design 2: Use of buccal canine retractors (Figure 3.5)

Indications

- Retraction of buccally displaced canines that are mesially tipped

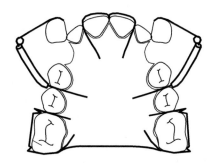

Please construct a URA to retract the upper canine teeth:

1. Buccal canine retractors UR3, UL3 – 0.5 mm hard ss wire with 0.7 mm internal diameter sleeve (also known as tubing)
2. Adams' clasps UR6, UL6 – 0.7 mm hard ss wire
3. Southend clasp UR1, UL1 – 0.7 mm hard ss wire
4. Baseplate saddled as indicated

Figure 3.5 Laboratory prescription for a URA to retract buccally placed upper permanent canine teeth.

Buccal canine retractors are rarely used now, as canines usually erupt buccally only if the arch is crowded. If the arch is crowded, then space will need to be created prior to alignment of the canines. As the canines erupt around the same time as the second premolars, the patient is likely to be in the permanent dentition and, therefore, fixed appliances following the extraction of first premolars is the preferred option in most cases.

Contra-indications

* Patients with a decreased buccal sulcus depth
  Rationale: The design of the spring means that it sits in the buccal sulcus. If there is inadequate sulcus depth the spring is more likely to cause ulceration in the buccal sulcus and, consequently, discomfort for the patient leading to an understandable lack of compliance.
* Canines are upright or are already distally tipped
  See above comments in relation to palatal finger springs.

Design features (see Figure 3.5)

Active: Buccal canine retractors on the upper permanent canine teeth (0.5 mm wire sleeved in ss tubing with an interior diameter of 0.7 mm).

Retention: Adams' clasps on upper first permanent molars (0.7 mm hard ss wire) and a Southend clasp on upper permanent central incisors (0.7 mm hard ss wire).

Anchorage: Care needs to be taken with the anchorage in this case. The reaction to the force applied to the canine teeth to move them distally will be movement of the anchor teeth and the appliance mesially. Canines are large teeth and need more force to move them than the incisors. Therefore, anchorage must be monitored carefully to ensure that it is not lost.

Baseplate: If the overbite is increased, then an FABP may be included as appropriate in order to decrease it.

Colleting distal to the upper lateral incisors and mesial to the upper first premolars needs to remain in place to prevent any unwanted drifting of these teeth.

Fitting and activation: See Chapter 4.

Design 3: Use of orthodontic screws (Figure 3.6)

Indications

* For distal movement of blocks of teeth

For example, slight shortage of space (2–3 mm) for alignment of an upper or lower second premolar tooth due to mesial migration

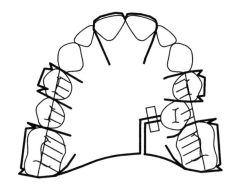

Please construct a URA to distalise UL6:

1. Orthodontic screw positioned as shown (note the angle – the screw should be drawn at an angle so that the UL6 is moved buccally *and* distally)

2. Adams' clasps UR6, UL6 – 0.7 mm hard ss wire

3. Adams' clasps UR4, UL4 – 0.7 mm hard ss wire

4. Southend clasp UR1, UL1 – 0.7 mm hard ss wire

5. ½ occlusal coverage posterior capping

6. Baseplate split as shown

Figure 3.6 Laboratory prescription for a URA to distalise UL6.

of the first molar on that side following early loss of the second primary molar.

Rationale: The advantage of using a screw in this situation is that the teeth that are being moved can also be included as part of the retention for the appliance.

Contra-indications

* More than 2–3 mm of space is required
* Space is required bilaterally

Rationale: Both the above situations will put too much stress on the anchorage, usually resulting in an increase in overjet (if used in the upper arch). This may be overcome by moving the buccal teeth on one side and then moving the buccal teeth on the other side. However, there are far more efficient methods of achieving this, e.g. extra-oral traction (headgear), which are largely outside the scope of this book and should not be undertaken by someone without the appropriate postgraduate training (see Chapter 10).

Design features of a URA to recreate space for UL5 by distalising UL6 (see Figure 3.6)

Active: Orthodontic expansion screw positioned so as to open space between UL5 and UL6.

Retention: Adams' clasps on the upper first permanent molars (0.7 mm hard ss wire) and upper first premolars (0.7 mm hard ss wire).
    Southend clasp on the upper central incisors (0.7 mm hard ss mm).

Anchorage: Care needs to be taken with the anchorage in this case. The reaction to the force applied to the buccal teeth to move them distally will be movement of the anchor teeth and the appliance mesially. If this occurs, then the buccal segment relationship on the contralateral side will be disrupted, becoming more Class II, and there will be an increase in overjet.

Baseplate: The acrylic should be sectioned to allow the buccal segment to distalise. Also, it is often helpful in cases where the upper and lower teeth are well inter-digitated to include thin posterior capping to free up the occlusion and so allow unencumbered tooth movement.

Fitting and activation: See Chapter 4.

Design features of a LRA to recreate space for LR5 by distalising LR6 (see Figure 3.7)

Active: Orthodontic expansion screw is positioned so as to open space between LR5 and LR6.

Retention: Adams' clasps on lower first permanent molars (0.7 mm hard ss wire) and lower first premolars (0.7 mm hard ss wire); labial bow around the lower labial segment (0.7 mm hard ss).

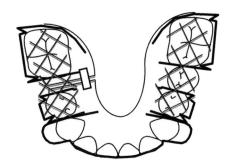

Please construct a LRA to distalise LR6:

1. Orthodontic screw positioned as shown

2. Adams' clasps LR6, LL6 – 0.7 mm hard ss wire

3. Adams' clasps LR4, LL4 – 0.7 mm hard ss wire

4. Labial bow LR3–LL3 – 0.7 mm hard ss wire

5. ½ occlusal coverage posterior capping

6. Baseplate split as shown

Figure 3.7 Laboratory prescription for a LRA to distalise LR6 to allow eruption of LR5.

Anchorage: Care needs to be taken with the anchorage in this case. The reaction to the force applied to the buccal teeth to move them distally will be movement of the anchor teeth and the appliance mesially. If this occurs, then the buccal segment relationship on the contra-lateral side will be disrupted, becoming more Class III. Also, the lower incisors may become excessively proclined, jeopardising the integrity of the periodontium and potentially resulting in a Class III incisor relationship. This is especially so if the second molar teeth have already erupted, as the lower first and second molars have a significantly greater resistance to movement than the lower labial segment due to the difference in root surface area (see Figure 2.1).

Baseplate: The acrylic should be sectioned to allow the buccal segment to distalise. Also, it is often helpful in cases where the upper and lower teeth are well inter-digitated to include thin (1.5 mm) posterior capping to free up the occlusion and so allow unencumbered tooth movement.

Fitting and activation: See Chapter 4

Moving teeth labially

URAs are extremely useful for pushing teeth labially to correct anterior crossbites. Anterior crossbites are often associated with a forward displacement of the mandible on closure. URAs may be used to push single teeth or blocks of teeth 'over the bite'. The main advantage of this over the use of fixed appliances is that posterior bite blocks (posterior capping) may be incorporated to open the bite and so remove any hindrance to tooth movement by the lower teeth. The spring design varies depending on whether the tooth to be moved is an incisor or a tooth in the buccal segment: Z-springs are used for incisors and canines; T-springs are used for premolars and molars, as these springs fit the palatal surfaces best. When blocks of teeth are being moved, expansion screws are used. If

two adjacent incisor teeth are to be moved labially, then a 'double Z-spring' or re-curved spring may be used, providing the direction of movement is the same for both teeth.

If the anterior crossbite is associated with an anterior displacement of the mandible on closure, then once the crossbite has been corrected and the displacement has been eliminated, the overjet will increase. The patient and parents/guardian must be warned of this likelihood.

Occasionally it can be difficult or impossible to detect a displacement on closure, as the patient may be so used to avoiding the premature occlusal contact. If there is some wear of the incisor edge, this may suggest a displacement exists, but, if in doubt, it is probably best to assume there is no displacement on closure for the reason illustrated below.

Design 1: Use of Z-springs (Figure 3.8)

Indications

* Pushing single teeth labially (proclining them) to correct anterior crossbites in a patient who has an anterior displacement of the mandible on closure and/or there is gingival recession on the labial aspect of the lower tooth involved in the crossbite

This pattern of gingival recession is very commonly a consequence of an anterior crossbite (Figure 3.9). Therefore, if recession is present in a young patient, then the presence of a mandibular displacement should be assumed until proven otherwise.

Rationale: Z-springs may be used for correction of crossbites on any of the incisors. Central incisors may be in crossbite in patients with a Class III tendency, while crossbites on lateral incisors are often associated with crowding. In this situation, it may be necessary to extract the primary canine teeth bilaterally to provide space into which to move the lateral incisor teeth. If the primary canines are removed to allow movement of the lateral incisor(s), then the patient

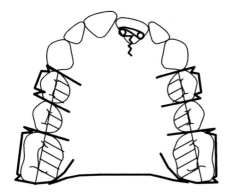

Please construct a URA to procline UL1:

1. Z-spring UL1 – 0.5 mm hard ss wire

2. Adams' clasps UR6, UL6 – 0.7 mm hard ss wire

3. Adams' clasps UR4, UL4 – 0.7 mm hard ss wire

4. ½ occlusal coverage posterior capping

Figure 3.8 Laboratory prescription for a URA to procline UL1 to correct an anterior crossbite.

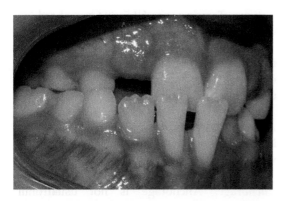

Figure 3.9 Marked recession of the labial gingivae on the lower incisors and proclination of these teeth. This is due to the effects of the upper incisors occluding lingual to the lower incisors as a consequence of an anterior mandibular displacement from an edge-to-edge incisor relationship.

and parents/guardian should be warned that the crowding will relocate to the canine region and further orthodontic treatment with fixed appliances may be required at a later date.

Contra-indications

- There is no displacement of the mandible
  Rationale: If a crossbite exists with the mandible in the RCP, then a significant amount of tooth movement will be required to correct it. If a URA is used to tip the tooth, the root apex will remain in its original position, leading to excessive proclination. In these situations it is preferable to use fixed appliances in the permanent dentition because fixed appliances will be able to move the whole tooth labially by bodily movement.
- There is minimal or no overbite at the start of treatment
  Rationale: When teeth are proclined by tipping, there is also a relative intrusion (see Chapter 2). This decreases the overbite. An adequate overbite at the end of treatment is essential to maintain the crossbite correction. Therefore, in situations where there is only a very small overbite or an anterior open bite at the start of treatment, there is likely to be significant relapse of the orthodontic tooth movements.
- The teeth to be moved labially are already proclined
  Rationale: Any further proclination through tipping will lead to non-axial loading of the tooth during biting, which is potentially detrimental to the tooth and the supporting tissues. Furthermore, teeth that are very proclined are also very unaesthetic.

Design features of a URA to procline UL1 (see Figure 3.8)

Active: Z-spring UL1 (0.5 mm wire).

Retention: Adams' clasps on upper first permanent molars (0.7 mm hard ss wire) and upper first premolars (0.7 mm hard ss wire) or upper first primary molars (0.6 mm hard ss wire).

Anchorage: Anchorage is not usually a problem in these types of cases as the reaction to the force used to procline UL1 will be in a distal direction and the anchor unit will be large as all the other teeth will be included.

Baseplate: Posterior capping should be included to disengage the occlusion and so allow uninhibited labial movement of UL1. If the overbite is increased and only one tooth needs to be moved labially, a flat anterior biteplane may be included instead. The use of posterior capping often increases the overbite as it allows further eruption of the incisor teeth that are not being restrained by the appliance (usually the lower incisors).

Fitting and activation: See Chapter 4.

Design 2: Use of T-springs (Figure 3.10)

Indications

- Correcting a crossbite on a single premolar or molar tooth

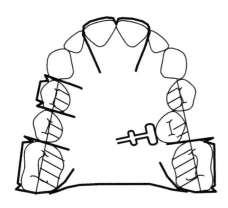

Please construct a URA to push UL5 buccally:

1. T-spring UL5 -0.6 mm hard ss wire

2. Adams' clasps UR6, UL6 – 0.7 mm hard ss wire

3. Adams' clasps UR4 – 0.7 mm hard ss wire

4. Southend clasp UR1, UL1 – 0.7 mm hard ss wire

5. ½ posterior capping relieved around UL5

Figure 3.10 Laboratory prescription for a URA to push a palatally-displaced UL5 buccally.

For example, an in-standing second premolar tooth which may be causing a lateral displacement of the mandible.

Contra-indications

- Tooth is buccally tipped already (see contra-indications for the use of Z-springs)
- There is minimal cuspal interlocking or a frank lateral open bite
- There is insufficient space to move the tooth buccally

Rationale: In this situation, correction of the crossbite will relapse as contact between the upper and lower teeth is essential to ensure stability. In addition, if there is insufficient space to move the tooth buccally, then of course the tooth will not move.

Design features of a URA to push UL5 buccally (see Figure 3.10)

Active: T-spring on UL5 (0.6 mm hard ss wire).

Retention: Adams' clasps on upper first permanent molars (0.7 mm hard ss wire) and upper right first premolar (0.7 mm wire).
Southend clasp on UR1, UL1 (0.7 mm wire). A clasp is not incorporated on UL4 to limit interference with tooth movement from the wire components.

Anchorage: Anchorage is not usually a problem in these types of cases as the reaction to the force used to push UL5 buccally will be to push all the other teeth that are contained in the anchor unit to the opposite side of the mouth. The anchor unit will be large as all the other teeth and the palatal vault will be included.

Baseplate: Depending on the overbite, the occlusion may be disengaged either by using a flat anterior biteplane or posterior capping that is relieved around UL5, both buccally and occlusally, so as not to inhibit tooth movement.

Fitting and activation: See Chapter 4.

Design 3: Use of an expansion screw to move a block of teeth labially (Figure 3.11)

Indications

* Correction of anterior crossbite involving three or four incisor teeth

Rationale: In this case, careful assessment needs to be undertaken prior to considering treatment due to the likelihood of an underlying Class III skeletal discrepancy. Treatment should only be undertaken with a URA in the following circumstances:

* There is a mandibular displacement anteriorly from an edge-to-edge incisor relationship

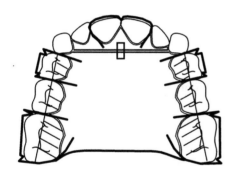

Please construct a URA to procline UR12, UL12:

1. Orthodontic screw in position shown

2. Adams' clasps UR6, UL6 – 0.7 mm hard ss wire

3. Adams' clasps URD, ULD – 0.6 mm hard ss wire

4. Southend clasp UR1, UL1 – 0.7 mm hard ss wire

5. ½ occlusal coverage posterior capping

6. Baseplate split as shown

Figure 3.11 Laboratory prescription for a URA to procline the upper incisor teeth to correct an anterior crossbite.

* There is an adequate overbite to ensure stability of correction
* The upper incisors are *not* proclined/the lower incisors are *not* retroclined. Both of these indicate dental compensation for a significant underlying skeletal discrepancy.

Contra-indications

* There is no displacement of the mandible

Rationale: If a crossbite exists on three or more incisor teeth with the mandible in the RCP, then it is possible that a significant Class III skeletal discrepancy underlies the malocclusion. Future growth during the adolescent growth spurt is likely to worsen the malocclusion and cause the relapse of any correction of the crossbite undertaken in the mixed dentition.

* There is minimal or no overbite at the start of treatment (see above, labial movement of single teeth).
* The teeth to be moved labially are already proclined (see above, labial movement of single teeth).
* The teeth to be moved require labial movement but in different directions. A screw appliance will move the block of teeth in one direction only, which may not be appropriate.

Design features of a URA to correct an anterior crossbite of the upper incisor teeth (see Figure 3.11)

Active: Orthodontic expansion screw.

Retention: Adams' clasps on upper first permanent molars (0.7 mm hard ss wire) ± on upper first premolars (0.7 mm hard ss wire) or upper first primary molars (0.6 mm hard ss wire).

Southend clasp on UR1, UL1 (0.7 mm hard ss wire) or labial bow fitted on UR12, UL12 (0.7 mm hard ss wire).

Anchorage: Anchorage is not usually a problem in these types of cases as the reaction to
the force used to procline UR12, UL12 will be
in a distal direction. The anchor unit will be
large as all the other teeth and the palatal vault
will be included. However, as the patient may
have an underlying skeletal Class III, any distal
movement of the anchor teeth should be
avoided.

Baseplate: Split transversely to allow anterior
movement of incisor teeth.

½ occlusal coverage posterior capping to
disengage occlusion and allow free movement
of upper teeth. Posterior capping will encourage the incisors to erupt and so will increase
the overbite. This can often be beneficial in
terms of stability at the end of treatment.

Fitting and activation: See Chapter 4.

Reduction of overbite

Removable appliances are the most efficient
method of overbite reduction, especially in
individuals who are still growing. Increased
overbites are often caused by an increased
curve of Spee in the lower arch and need to be
reduced prior to overjet reduction. Also, they
may be reduced to assist with restorative
requirements for the anterior dentition.

URAs that incorporate FABPs correct the
overbite by having the lower incisors in contact
with the biteplane, but the buccal segments out
of contact. This allows the lower buccal segment
teeth to erupt, which they do until they contact
the upper buccal segment teeth, which are prevented from erupting by the presence of the
URA. This flattens the curve of Spee and
decreases the overbite (Figure 3.12).

FABPs may be incorporated as required into
most designs of removable appliances, apart
from screw appliances to correct crossbites on
three or four incisor teeth. They can also be
used purely as a biteplane before or during
treatment with fixed appliances.

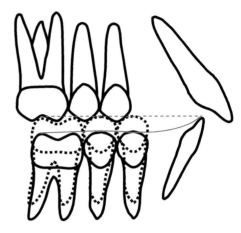

Figure 3.12   Diagrammatic representation of overbite reduction using an FABP. The dotted outlines
indicate the eruption of the lower buccal teeth following disengagement of the occlusion with the biteplane.
Note how this allows the increased curve of Spee
(solid red line) to be levelled (dashed red line). The
biteplane should create 2–3 mm of separation of the
buccal teeth. The lower buccal teeth erupt into this space.

Design: Flat anterior biteplane (Figure 3.13)

Indications

• Reduction of increased overbite

Contra-indications

• Caution should be exercised in patients who
have increased lower anterior face height
and increased Frankfort–mandibular planes
angle (FMPA) as a further increase in face
height due to eruption of the molar teeth
would be undesirable
• Rarely, an increased overbite can be due
to the upper incisors having overerupted
rather than an increased curve of Spee in the
lower arch. An FABP in this situation may
not be appropriate

*Design features of a URA to reduce
increased overbite (see Figure 3.13)*

Active: Flat anterior biteplane.

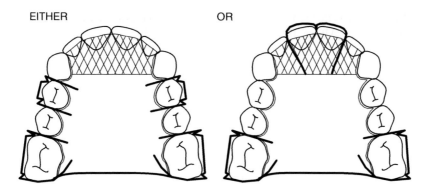

EITHER   OR

Please construct a URA to reduce the overbite:

   1. Adams' clasps UR6, UL6 – 0.7 mm hard ss wire

   2. Adams' clasps UR4, UL4 – 0.7 mm hard ss wire

       or

   Southend clasp UR1, UL1 – 0.7 mm hard sss wire

   3. Baseplate – please extend posteriorly by 10 mm (OJ 8 mm) and cover 2/3
      of the height of the upper central incisor crowns

Figure 3.13 Laboratory prescription for a URA with a flat anterior biteplane to reduce an increased overbite.

Retention: Adams' clasps on upper first permanent molars (0.7 mm hard ss wire) and upper first premolars (0.7 mm hard ss wire) or upper first primary molars (0.6 mm hard ss wire) *or* (if primary molars are exfoliating and permanent successors are not yet erupted) Adams' clasps on upper first permanent molars (0.7 mm hard ss wire) and Southend clasp on upper central incisors (0.7 mm hard ss wire).

Anchorage: No active tooth movement with springs or screws, therefore anchorage is not an issue.

Baseplate: It is essential that the laboratory technician is provided with the appropriate information to allow the biteplane to have adequate height and depth. Therefore, if only an upper working model is provided to the technician, the prescription must include a measurement of the overjet and also an indication of where the biteplane should finish in relation to the height of the palatal surfaces of the upper central incisors. The biteplane should extend posteriorly by approximately 2–3 mm greater than the measurement of the overjet. Bearing in mind that the overjet is measured from the labial surface of the lower incisor to the upper incisor tip, this should provide 4–5 mm of acrylic posterior to the lower incisor tips, which should be adequate to prevent the lower incisors occluding behind the biteplane. Without a measurement of the overjet, it is possible, in cases with an increased overjet, that the biteplane will not be extended far enough posteriorly, allowing the lower incisors to occlude behind it. This will have no effect on the overbite, or may even increase it, but may restrict growth of the mandible. If an indication of height is not provided, it may be that there will be inadequate separation of the posterior teeth, necessitating addition of acrylic to the biteplane after a short period of time. Alternatively, if the biteplane is too high and the separation is too great, this may affect compliance.

If the upper second permanent molars have already erupted, then it is essential to incorporate occlusal rests on these teeth into the appliance design in order to prevent them from over-erupting. Upper 7s over-erupt very quickly, given the opportunity, and great care must always be taken to prevent this from happening, as a marked anterior open bite will result. An example of the laboratory prescription is given in Figure 6.20.

Fitting and activation: See Chapter 4.

Reducing an overjet

Historically, URAs were used for overjet reduction, following the extraction of the upper first premolars and retraction of the canines. The active components were either labial bows (short or long reverse loop) or Robert's retractors.

Unfortunately, reduction of an overjet by this method often resulted in changing a Class II division 1 malocclusion into a Class II division 2 malocclusion due to the fact that removable appliances are only able to tip teeth. This often looked not only dentally unattractive (one malocclusion having been swapped for another), but also, if teeth had been extracted in the lower arch, resulted in a highly unattractive facial appearance. At the end of treatment by this method, the upper incisors were often not under the control of the lower lip, which is essential for stability following the correction of large overjets. This led to relapse as the lower lip proclined the upper incisors again; not only did the upper incisors return to their original position, but they were now also spaced as first premolars had been removed. In some cases, the teeth may also have been damaged, potentially making further (re)-treatment difficult if not impossible.

Most patients with an increased overjet require bodily movement of the upper incisors during overjet reduction. Therefore, in modern orthodontics, fixed appliances are the treatment method of choice in these cases and removable appliances should not be used.

There is one specific situation in which a very small increase in overjet may be corrected using removable appliances, as described below.

Design: A URA to retrocline upper incisors, reducing overjet and eliminating spacing (see Figure 3.14)

Indications

The indications for this type of appliance are very specific:

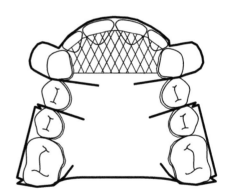

Please construct a URA to reduce the overbite and overjet:

1. Labial bow UR321, UL123 – 0.7 mm hard ss wire

2. Double Adams' clasps UR65, UL56 – 0.7 mm hard ss wire

3. Baseplate – please extend posteriorly by 7 mm (OJ 5 mm) and cover ½ of the height of the upper central incisor crowns

Figure 3.14 Laboratory prescription for a URA to reduce overbite and then close mild anterior spacing ± reducing a slightly increased overjet.

- The upper incisors are spaced and only *slightly* proclined
- The overjet is only very slightly increased (overjet no more than 5 mm)
- The overbite is incomplete.

This situation may be seen in a patient who has had orthodontic treatment to reduce a large overjet, but who has stopped wearing the retainer. However, if the previous treatment has relapsed to some degree, it is unlikely that the teeth were placed in a position of soft tissue balance. The patient should be warned that once the spaces/overjet have been reduced again, they will need to wear some form of retaining device indefinitely.

Contra-indications

- A larger overjet requiring bodily movement of the teeth to achieve a stable and aesthetic result

Design features of a URA to retrocline upper incisors, reducing overjet and eliminating spacing (see Figure 3.14)

Active: Labial bow (0.7 mm hard ss wire) from UR3 to UL3.

Retention: Double clasps on upper first permanent molars and upper second premolars (0.7 mm hard ss wire). This brings the posterior retention as far forward as possible without interfering with the labial bow.

Anchorage: Care must be taken with activation of the labial bow as the equal and opposite reaction will be to bring the appliance and the anchor teeth more anteriorly, disrupting the molar relationship.

Baseplate: If the overbite is complete, then a small flat anterior biteplane may be included to reduce the overbite and so allow retroclination of the upper incisors.

Fitting and activation: See Chapter 4.

Other individual tooth movements: Extrusion of incisors

It is very rare for central incisors not to erupt into the correct position unless there has been a specific impedance to their eruption. Of course, they may be intruded as a consequence of dento-alveolar trauma. Thus, children with intruded incisors are usually seen by orthodontic specialists, often in conjunction with paediatric dentists. However, under the guidance of a specialist, there is no reason why extrusion of incisors cannot be undertaken by non-specialists once the eruptive path is clear and/or the tooth has been 'passed fit' for orthodontic tooth movement, as long as they have the necessary attachments to bond to the labial surface of the tooth to be extruded.

Design: A URA to extrude an intruded UL1 (see Figures 3.15 and 3.16)

Indications

- Extrusion of an incisor that has failed to erupt sufficiently following the removal of an impedance to eruption (e.g. ankylosed primary tooth; supernumerary) in a patient who is in the mixed dentition
- Re-extrusion of a tooth that has been intruded as a consequence of trauma in a patient in the mixed dentition

This assumes that there is no pathology associated with the root of the traumatised tooth

Contra-indications

- Clinical and/or radiographic evidence of root pathology (resorption, periapical radiolucency)
- The tooth is ankylosed
- The tooth is palatally positioned

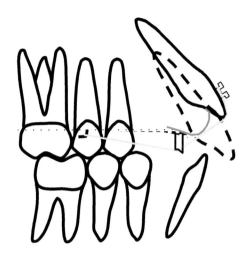

Figure 3.15 Diagram to show positioning of a hook and 'goalpost' in a URA to extrude upper incisor. Note the position of the elastic band (yellow line) in relation to the gingivae (pink outline). Stretching the elastic band over the 'goalpost' keeps it away from the gingivae and prevents it from causing trauma to the gingivae.

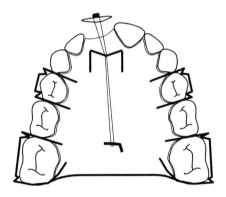

Please construct a URA to allow extrusion of UR1:

1. "Goalpost" positioned behind upper incisors – 3 mm overjet and average overbite

2. Hook positioned in baseplate opposite first permanent molars, facing distally

3. Adams' clasps UR6, UL6 – 0.7 mm hard ss wire

4. Adams' clasps UR4, UL4 – 0.7 mm hard ss wire

5. Baseplate

Figure 3.16 Laboratory prescription for a URA to extrude UR1. Note the position of the hook and 'goalpost'.

Rationale: The force vectors generated by the use of elastic bands to extrude the tooth mean that the tooth is pulled palatally at the same time as being extruded and, therefore, may induce a crossbite.

- If the patient is in the permanent dentition, then a fixed appliance would be more appropriate.

Design features of a URA to extrude an incisor (see Figure 3.16)

Active: Intra-oral elastic band stretched from attachment bonded to labial surface of incisor to a hook positioned on the baseplate.

Retention: Adams' clasps on upper first permanent molars (0.7 mm hard ss wire) and upper first premolars (0.7 mm wire) or upper first primary molars (0.6 mm wire).

Anchorage: With this type of tooth movement, anchorage is required to prevent an upward movement of the appliance and intrusion of the teeth incorporated into the anchorage unit. Although the palatal vault should provide plenty of anchorage against an upward movement, the position of the arrowheads on the clasps should be checked carefully at each visit to ensure that they are not becoming sub-gingival.

Baseplate: Although the description of the baseplate usually refers to the use of acrylic, in this situation two important wire-work features are incorporated into the baseplate: the 'hook' to which the elastic band is attached and the 'goalpost' (a 'goalpost'-shaped piece of wire). It is positioned anteriorly in the baseplate (avoiding occlusal interference with the lower incisors) and the elastic band is stretched over it. This lifts the elastic band away from the mucosa/gingivae and prevents trauma from the elastic band (Figure 3.15). A notch in the 'cross-bar' is useful to aid location of the elastic band (this is also illustrated in the laboratory prescription of Figure 3.16).

Fitting and activation: See Chapter 4.

Space maintainers

Space maintainers are extremely useful in severely crowded malocclusions in which teeth may be impacted due to the lack of space to accommodate them in the arch. They may be used prior to the use of fixed appliances or, if the malocclusion would be very mild once the impacted teeth have erupted, then a space maintainer may be the only appliance necessary. The ideal time for this treatment is in the late mixed dentition, when the permanent dentition is awaited prior to the start of fixed appliance treatment. Using a space maintainer to hold space following the extraction of permanent teeth to allow other teeth space to erupt, decreases the amount of tooth movement required with fixed appliances. Allowing the teeth to erupt naturally rather than being exposed and aligned improves the gingival condition at the end of treatment, because they erupt through attached mucosa.

Unfortunately, many cases that are suitable for space maintainers have impacted teeth due to mesial drift of the first permanent molars following early loss of the primary molars, most often due to caries. It is imperative that the circumstances that caused the loss of the primary molars, e.g. cariogenic diet and poor oral hygiene, have been rectified prior to use of a space maintainer.

With all removable appliances, the appliance should be fitted *prior* to the extraction of teeth. This is especially the case with space maintainers as in severely crowded malocclusions, space may be lost by unwanted tooth movement very quickly after the extraction of teeth.

Under no circumstances should the extraction of sound permanent teeth to allow the eruption of impacted teeth be undertaken without first seeking the advice of a specialist orthodontist.

3.7.1 Design: Space maintainer (Figure 3.17)

Indications

- Maintenance of space following extraction of primary or permanent tooth/teeth to allow eruption of permanent teeth/impacted permanent teeth
- To maintain the leeway space following the extraction/exfoliation of a primary molar tooth to enable subsequent alignment of mildly crowded arches with fixed appliances without the need for any further space creation by extractions or enamel reduction

Contra-indications

- Patients who have not improved their diet or oral hygiene
- Young patients in whom a space maintainer would need to be worn for a prolonged period of time. This only serves to reduce co-operation with any subsequent treatment with fixed appliances. It also risks damaging the teeth (e.g. should caries occur), which can then completely compromise the later, definitive treatment
- Maintaining insufficient space. There is never any point in maintaining insufficient space

Design features of a URA to maintain space for the eruption of crowded permanent canine teeth following extraction of upper first premolars (see Figure 3.17)

Active: None, the appliance is passive.

Retention: Adams' clasps on upper first permanent molars (0.7 mm hard ss wire) and Southend clasp on upper central incisors (0.7 mm hard ss wire).

or

Double clasps on upper first permanent molars and upper second primary molars (0.7 mm hard ss wire), and Southend clasp on upper central incisors (0.7 mm hard ss wire). The double

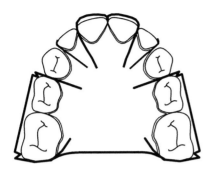

Please construct a URA to maintain the space for the unerupted upper canine teeth following the extraction of the upper first premolars:

    1. Double clasps UR6E, ULE6 – 0.7 mm hard ss wire

    2. Southend clasp UR1, UL1 – 0.7 mm

    3. Stops distal to UR2, UL2 – 0.6 mm

    4. Baseplate

Figure 3.17 Laboratory prescription for a URA to maintain space for the eruption of the upper permanent canine teeth following the extraction of the upper first premolar teeth.

clasps act as a 'stop' mesial to the second primary molars to prevent mesial drift of these teeth into the space vacated by extraction of the upper first premolars.

Also, wire stops may be added to prevent the teeth mesial/distal to the space from drifting into the space once the extractions have been undertaken.

Anchorage: No active tooth movement, therefore anchorage is not an issue.

Baseplate: Colleting distal to the upper lateral incisors and mesial to the upper second primary molars needs to remain in place to prevent any unwanted drifting of these teeth, especially if no wire-work to prevent this happening has been incorporated into the design.

If the overbite is increased, then an FABP may be included as appropriate in order to decrease it.

Design features of a LRA to maintain space for the eruption of lower second premolar teeth and the alignment of lower first premolar teeth following extraction of lower second primary molars (see Figure 3.18)

The loss of the lower second primary molar teeth, after a space maintainer has been fitted, provides not only enough space for the lower second premolar teeth to erupt, but also up to 2 mm of crowding of the lower first premolar teeth to be corrected, due to the 2.5 mm of leeway space available on each side of the lower arch.

Active: None, the appliance is passive.

Retention: Adams' clasps on lower first permanent molars (0.7 mm hard ss wire) and labial bow around lower labial segment (0.7 mm wire).

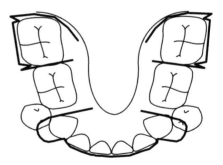

Please construct a LRA to maintain the space for the unerupted lower second premolar teeth following the extraction of the lower second primary molars:

    1. Adams' clasps LR6, LL6 – 0.7 mm hard ss wire

    2. Labial bow LR321, LL123 – 0.7 mm hard ss wire

    3. Baseplate

Figure 3.18 Laboratory prescription for a LRA to maintain space for the eruption of the lower second premolar teeth following the extraction of the lower second primary molar teeth.

Anchorage: No active tooth movement, therefore anchorage not an issue.

Baseplate: Colleting distal to the lower first premolars needs to be removed to allow some distal movement of these teeth. If these teeth are positioned buccally, then some limited trimming of the acrylic on the lingual aspect of the first premolars will allow them to drift lingually as well as distally as they align.

Basic errors

Although following the principles in this book should enable you to avoid errors in design, here we highlight three very common errors that prevent the appliance from working:

- Incorporating a Southend clasp on UR1, UL1 as anterior retention when the active component is a midline expansion screw.
- Incorporating a Southend clasp or fitted labial bow as anterior retention around a tooth that requires labial movement with a Z-spring.
- Incorporating a labial bow as anterior retention whose fly-overs lie distal to a tooth that is being moved distally with a palatal finger spring.

When these designs are drawn onto the prescription card, it should become apparent immediately that the retentive components are preventing tooth movement or activation of the active components. Repositioning of retentive components or different active and/or retentive components should be chosen instead to ensure that the appliance will be able to move the teeth as appropriate.

Summary

The appliance designs described in this chapter include those employed most commonly to achieve the desired tooth movements. Obviously, they do not cover the full range of possibilities and it may be necessary to adapt appliances, always using the principles described. Whilst it may be possible to use several appliances to undertake a sequence of movements, multiple tooth movements are invariably far more satisfactorily carried out using fixed appliances. However, if the principles of appliance design described in Chapter 2 are adhered to, then it should be possible to design an appliance for a range of interceptive orthodontic problems, choosing the components as appropriate.

Fitting and Activating Removable Appliances

4

The fitting and activation of upper removable appliances (URAs) should be a relatively straightforward and quick procedure, even for the less experienced, if the steps in this chapter are followed and you develop a routine with which you become familiar.

It is imperative that you become very adept at fitting and activating appliances as a poorly fitting appliance will provide the patient with an excuse not to wear it and, worse, an incorrectly activated appliance may have a significant detrimental effect on the malocclusion.

Learning outcomes

At the end of this chapter you should have knowledge and understanding of:

- What to check prior to fitting the appliance
- The advice that should be provided to the patient prior to fitting
- How to fit the appliance, what to check for and how to improve the fit of ill-fitting appliances

---

- How to increase the retention of the appliance
- How to activate the appliance
- How to instruct the patient on the insertion and removal of the appliance
- The instructions and advice that should be given to the patient/parent/guardian before they leave the surgery

When the URA arrives from the laboratory

The impressions and the design prescription for the construction of the URA will have been sent to a dental laboratory technician. It is important that a laboratory technician who is familiar with making orthodontic appliances is used. This may mean using a different laboratory from where your restorative work is produced.

Also, appliances should routinely be fitted within 2 weeks of the impression being taken to minimise the risk of the appliance not fitting

---

Orthodontic Retainers and Removable Appliances: Principles of Design and Use, First Edition.
Friedy Luther and Zararna Nelson-Moon.
© 2013 Friedy Luther and Zararna Nelson-Moon. Published 2013 by Blackwell Publishing Ltd.

due to tooth movement/eruption in the intervening time.

As with all laboratory-produced work, the following should be checked:

- That you have the correct appliance for that particular patient
- That the appliance has been made accurately to the prescription
- That there are no sharp spicules of acrylic on the fit surface or polished surfaces
- That the tag ends of the various wire components do not come through the acrylic on the fit surface
- That the active components, screws and springs move freely, and there are no spicules of acrylic preventing movement.

Obviously, if the appliance has not been made to the prescription requested, it will need to be re-made. It may be possible to re-use the working model, but this will need to be inspected carefully and, if in doubt, it is better to take another impression.

Spicules of acrylic or sharp wires can easily be trimmed using a straight handpiece with an acrylic-trimming bur or green stone (Figure 4.1).

All active components need to be checked for movement. Palatal finger springs are most often restricted by spicules of acrylic. It is also important to ensure that the location holes for the key that turns the expansion screws are all free of plaster/acrylic and that the key can be located easily. It is sensible to check that the screw can be turned prior to demonstrating this to the patient as, occasionally, they can be quite stiff (see later for details and a demonstration of the activation of an expansion screw).

Advice to the patient prior to fitting

The majority of patients being treated with URAs in general dental practice will be young and having interceptive treatment. The fitting

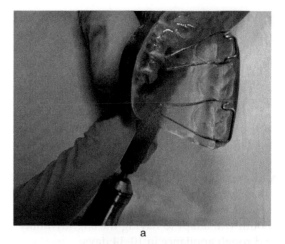

a

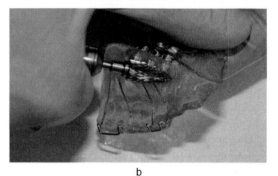

b

Figure 4.1 Spicules of acrylic or sharp wires can be trimmed using a straight handpiece with a green stone (a) or an acrylic-trimming bur (b), respectively.

of the appliance may be the first dental treatment that the patient has experienced, apart from having the impression taken. It is essential that the patient is advised appropriately and before any attempt is made to fit the appliance.

The patient should first be shown the appliance, both on and off the model, so they have some idea how the appliance will fit in their mouth. The patient should be warned that the appliance will:

- Feel very strange and very big when it is first fitted, 'a bit like having a football in your mouth'

- Make the patient lisp for the first few days, until the patient's tongue has become used to having an extra thickness on the palate
- Make the patient produce excess saliva for up to a couple of hours.

The patient should also be advised that instructions on how to insert and remove the appliance will be given once the fit of the appliance has been checked by the dentist; that they will become used to wearing the appliance after a few days (1–2 days normally if the URA is worn properly); and that the inside of their mouth will adapt to having the slightly bulky and rough appliance in 10–14 days.

Fitting the appliance and what to check for

Once the advice has been provided and the patient is happy to proceed, the appliance should be fitted:

- The appliance should be rotated into the patient's mouth, with the patient in the supine position.
- The appliance should be placed in position, then firmly seated with the tip of the finger against the palatal acrylic. A well-fitting appliance should elicit a click as it is seated in position and should not 'rock' when finger pressure is applied to each side of the baseplate.
- The retention of the appliance should be checked by trying to remove the appliance with downward pressure on the most posterior retentive components, usually Adams' clasps on the first permanent molars. A retentive device is one that requires firm finger pressure on the clasps to dislodge it. The patient should not be able to dislodge it with their tongue.
- All retentive components should be checked to ensure that they are positioned so that they engage the undercuts supra-gingivally and do not impinge on the gingivae. This is

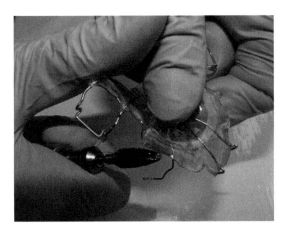

Figure 4.2 In this case, failure to remove the acrylic would prevent distal movement of UL3 by the palatal finger spring. Acrylic removal should be undertaken with an acrylic bur (as here) or greenstone on a straight handpiece.

especially the case for the arrowheads of the Adams' clasps.
- The baseplate should be checked for closeness of fit with the palate.
- The baseplate should also be checked to ensure that no acrylic will prevent the planned movement of teeth (Figure 4.2).
- If an anterior biteplane has been added to the appliance in order to reduce the overbite, then it is imperative that its height is sufficient to disengage the posterior occlusion by at least 2 mm. It is also necessary to ensure that there is even contact between the lower incisor and canine teeth with the biteplane as, if only one or two teeth are in contact, the full occlusal force will be transmitted through these teeth. This is potentially damaging to the teeth and will certainly make them very sore (Figure 4.3).
- If posterior capping has been included in the appliance to disengage the occlusion, then, as with the anterior biteplane, it is necessary to check that the posterior teeth contact the capping evenly in order to prevent differential eruption of the teeth not in contact and to limit discomfort from the appliance. It is

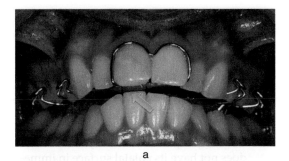

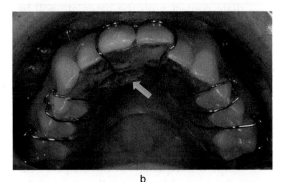

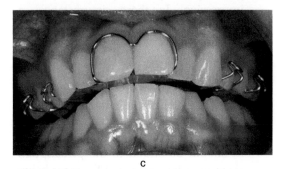

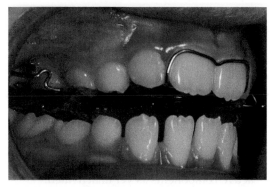

Figure 4.4   The posterior teeth contact the posterior capping evenly in order to prevent differential eruption of these teeth. The capping should provide enough separation of the anterior teeth to allow anterior crossbites to be corrected without the lower incisors preventing labial movement of the upper incisors, as shown here.

Trouble-shooting

An appliance that has been well made by an experienced technician will generally be able to be seated in the patient's mouth and is likely to require very little adjustment to make it fit really well. However, it is often necessary to increase the retention on the appliance, as it will become loose between the fitting and review appointments (see Chapter 5).

There are occasions when the appliance is unable to be seated or, if seated, is a poor fit. There are a number of reasons for this:

- Teeth have moved or erupted more since the impression was taken. This is more likely if there is a significant delay in fitting the appliance.
- The impression was distorted due to poor impression technique or being left too long under inappropriate conditions before being cast up.
- The appliance has been poorly made.

In many cases where the appliance does not fit straight away, it is possible to adjust the

Figure 4.3   Only one lower incisor (LR1) is in contact with this flat anterior biteplane (arrowed; a). It is necessary to ensure that there is even contact of at least three teeth with the biteplane. Therefore, the biteplane has been trimmed (arrowed; b) to bring three lower incisors into contact (c). Note that the biteplane is still active as shown by the posterior teeth being approximately 2 mm out of occlusion.

also essential to check that the capping separates the teeth enough to allow anterior crossbites to be corrected without the lower incisors preventing labial movement of the upper incisors (Figure 4.4).

appliance so that it fits or the fit becomes more acceptable. There are a series of steps that should be followed in order to determine the cause of the inadequate fit and how this can be rectified:

1. The active components should not be touched until the clinician has ensured that the appliance is a good fit. All removable appliances will be sent from the laboratory with the active components as yet unactivated.
2. The retentive components should be slackened so that there can be no hindrance to the fitting of the appliance by retentive components that are too tight.
3. If the appliance is still not seating adequately, then the cause is certain to be some aspect of the acrylic baseplate:
   ○ Check that the colleting around the palatal surfaces of the teeth fits snugly, but that none of the collets is preventing the appliance from seating. Also, acrylic that extends too far along the fly-overs on wire components can have the same affect (Figure 4.5). A thorough examina-

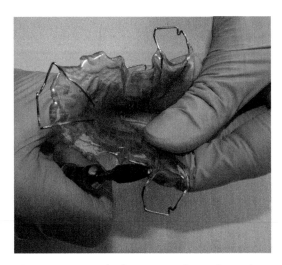

Figure 4.5 Acrylic that prevents the appliance from seating because it extends too far along the fly-overs on wire components should be removed, as shown here.

tion will usually reveal if one or more of the collets or the acrylic around a wire component needs to be relieved. If this is the case, then relieve one collet at a time, a little at a time, with the appliance out of the patient's mouth, using an acrylic-trimming bur in a straight handpiece. If there is over-zealous trimming of the collets/baseplate, then any tooth that does not have its palatal surface in immediate contact with the baseplate will be liable to drift palatally, especially if it is a tooth that has been clasped for retention purposes.
   ○ Once any problems associated with the colleting have been removed but the appliance still does not seat adequately, then, if there is no posterior capping incorporated into the appliance, the poor fit will be due to the baseplate not being adapted adequately to the shape of the palate, possibly due to distortion of the impression. In these circumstances a decision must be made by the clinician as to whether the appliance will become a tolerable fit once the retention has been increased again, or whether the fit is so inadequate that the appliance will have to be re-made. If the latter, then a new impression will need to be taken and the reasons why the initial appliance did not fit should be added to the prescription sheet in order to prevent the error being repeated.
   ○ However, if there is posterior capping incorporated into the appliance, the appliance may not seat because one of the teeth covered by the capping has erupted more or moved slightly since the impression was taken. It can sometimes be difficult to see exactly which tooth is causing the problem and, in these situations, it may be necessary to use denture relief cream on the fit surface in order that the area of initial contact between the teeth and baseplate may be identified and relieved.

○ Once the baseplate has been adjusted to seat adequately, the retention should be increased a little at a time until fitting the appliance elicits a sharp click when seated and requires firm downward pressure on the clasps to remove it.

○ Then, and only then, should the active components be activated.

Adjustment and/or activation of components

The correct adjustment of the retentive components and correct activation of the active components, in terms of both direction and force, are key to the success of a removable appliance.

Adjustment of retentive components

Adams' clasps

These are the main retentive components on all removable appliances and, as such, the success of the treatment depends on these being retentive enough to maintain the position of the appliance after activation. Many active components have a dislodging effect on the appliance once they have been activated and, without adequate retention, the appliance may not stay in the patient's mouth and, therefore, tooth movement will be much less effective.

Prior to adjustment, the operator must ensure that the appliance is seating adequately. Once this has been confirmed, the ease with which the appliance can be removed from the mouth should be checked. If the patient is able to dislodge the appliance easily with their tongue, or only minimal finger pressure is required, then the retention needs to be increased.

Prior to any adjustment, the correct positioning on the tooth of each part of the Adams' clasp must be established (Figure 4.6):

• The fly-overs should be as close to the contact points of the teeth as possible as they

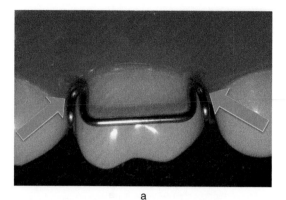

a

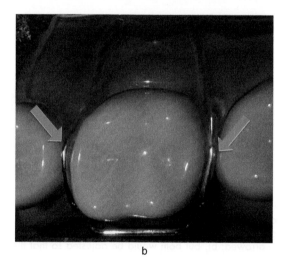

b

Figure 4.6 Design features of an Adams' clasp. Note the positioning of the arrowheads (arrowed; a) into the mesio- and disto-buccal undercuts of the first permanent molar, and the well-fitting fly-overs (arrowed; b) that sit well down into the embrasures to help avoid occlusal interferences with the lower arch.

crossover from the palatal acrylic to the buccal aspect of the tooth.

• The bridge should lie approximately two-thirds of the distance from the gingival margin to the cusp tips, and there should be a gap of no more than 1.5 mm between the bridge and the buccal surface of the tooth.

• The arrowheads should be positioned in the undercuts just above the gingival margins on the mesio-buccal and disto-buccal aspects of the crown.

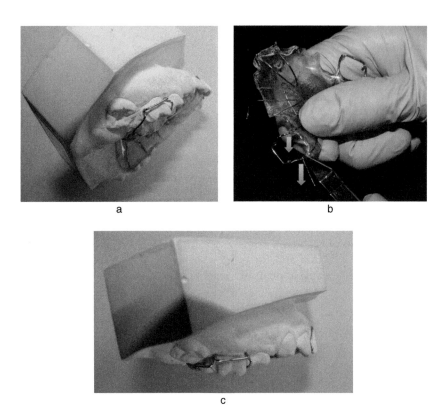

Figure 4.7 Adams' clasp adjustment of the fly-overs: when the arrowheads do not initially engage the under-cuts mesio- or disto-buccally (a), arrowed, then the fly-overs must be adjusted by bending them toward the gingivae where the wire exits the acrylic (b). Here the distal fly-over is being adjusted (direction of adjustment is arrowed; b), but both would be adjusted so that the undercuts are engaged as shown (c).

Of course, adjustment of one particular part of the Adams' clasp will affect the other aspects, so care must be taken with the adjustments and the position of every part of the crib checked after each adjustment. For example, adjustment to the fly-over to make it lie more closely against the contact points will move the arrow-heads closer to the gingival margin. It may also move the bridge away from the buccal surface of the tooth and closer to the buccal mucosa (Figure 4.7).

Adjusting a poorly fitting Adams' clasp to make it retentive can be frustrating and time-consuming for the inexperienced. Of course, there are limits to the amount of adjustment that can be carried out at the chairside and, if

the majority of appliances arriving back from the laboratory require significant adjustment, then this must be discussed with the laboratory technician or a different laboratory is used.

Once the position of all parts of the Adams' clasp has been checked, then the retention of the appliance should be re-checked. In theory, the correct positioning of the parts should ensure that the appliance has enough retention, but patient factors and the accuracy of the impression material need to be taken into account.

If the retention still needs to be increased, then this should now be a straightforward matter of adjusting the arrowheads (Figure 4.8). The beaks of the Adams' 64 pliers (also

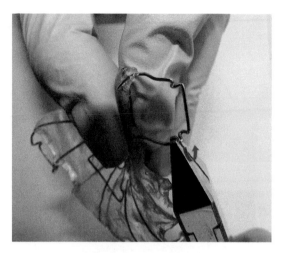

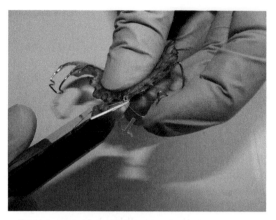

Figure 4.9 Tightening a Southend clasp: the pliers grip the clasp just where the wire exits the acrylic and finger pressure is applied to the vertical arms of the clasp so that each side is pushed firmly toward the baseplate (arrowed).

Figure 4.8 Where the arrowheads are engaging the undercuts, but retention still needs to be increased, both arrowheads may need to be adjusted, as shown here on the mesial arrowhead. The pliers grip the wire firmly and the appliance is turned so that each arrowhead more fully engages the undercut (arrowed). Care should be taken not to overtighten the appliance since the molars may become extruded; furthermore, the patient may struggle with excessive discomfort or difficulty fitting the appliance.

known as universal or simply 'Adams' pliers') should be placed just palatal to the arrowhead and a slight inward movement of the arrowheads made. Only very small adjustments should be made at this stage as the arrowheads are the most work-hardened part of the Adams' clasp and continual adjustment and readjustment will make them prone to fracture due to wire fatigue. Each Adams' clasp should be adjusted in turn. Enlisting the help of the patient is useful at this stage, as they will usually be able to tell you which clasps feel too tight and which too loose.

Retention is adequate when firm finger pressure on the clasps on both sides of the appliance is required to dislodge it.

Southend clasps

Southend clasps are used as retentive components in the anterior part of the mouth. They

engage the undercuts on the labial surface of the upper incisors, just incisal to the gingival margin. This undercut is more apparent in incisors that are normally inclined or proclined, and only limited retention can be gained from a Southend clasp placed on retroclined incisors.

Retention on a Southend clasp should not be adjusted until the appliance can be seated adequately and the retention on the Adams' clasps has been optimised. The positioning of the Southend clasp should be checked prior to any adjustment to ensure that the wire-work lies in the undercuts and does not impinge on the gingivae. The wire-work should contact the teeth.

The retention is increased by gripping the wire just as it emerges from the acrylic of the baseplate with the beaks of Adams' 64 pliers and applying gentle finger pressure to the Southend clasp to move it palatally and closer to the baseplate (Figure 4.9). This should be carried out at each of the two places where the wire emerges from the baseplate. It is important not to increase the retention so much that the patient has difficulty inserting or removing the appliance.

Labial bows

Labial bows may be used as retentive components anteriorly, although, as with Southend clasps, the retention gained from a labial bow is much better on normally inclined or proclined teeth and is minimal on retroclined teeth. The labial bow should lie in the middle third of the crowns of the incisor teeth with the U-loops adjacent to the canine teeth. It is important to check that the U-loops do not impinge on the gingivae or traumatise the buccal sulcus. The wire of the bow should contact as many of the incisor teeth as possible, depending upon how well aligned these teeth are. The acrylic of the baseplate should be in contact with the palatal surfaces of the teeth. The fly-overs should be in contact with the contact points between the upper canine and upper first premolar teeth (Figure 4.10).

Retention is increased by tightening the bow around the incisor teeth, so making it more difficult to dislodge on normally inclined or proclined teeth as the middle third of the tooth is lying on the arc of a smaller circle than the incisal edges of the teeth. The bow is tightened by contracting the U-loops. The beaks of the Adams' 64 pliers should be placed on either side of the vertical aspects of the U-loop and gentle pressure applied to bring the sides of the U-loop closer together (Figure 4.11). This action moves the bow palatally, but also incisally. If the bow now lies more incisally than the middle third of the crown of the teeth, then it needs to be adjusted to raise it up to its correct position again. This is achieved by gripping the base of the vertical arm of the U-loop that connects with the bow and applying gentle finger pressure to raise the bow (Figure 4.12). The same action should be carried out on the contralateral U-loop. The position of the bow should be checked again and the retention re-checked to ensure that raising the bow has not reduced the retention provided. Adequate retention is provided when there is obvious friction between the bow and the teeth when the bow

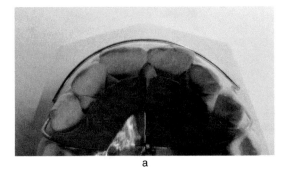

a

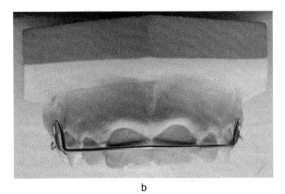

b

Figure 4.10 A well-fitting labial bow (a). Note its positioning, which should lie in the middle third of the upper incisor crowns (b); the wire-work forms a smooth curve contacting as much of the labial surfaces as possible (a); the U-loops lie adjacent to the canines and the fly-overs pass through the contact between the canines and the premolars.

is moved up and down, but it should not be so tight that it will not automatically position itself in the right place when the appliance is fully seated (Figure 4.12c).

Activation of active components

Z-springs

It is difficult to over-activate a Z-spring, mainly because it is extremely difficult to seat the appliance if the spring has been over-activated.

As a general rule, the Z-spring should be activated until the free arm lies just below the

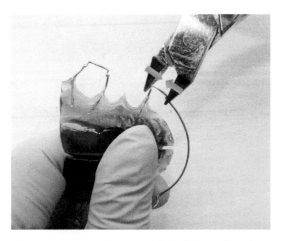

Figure 4.11 Tightening a labial bow: the pliers squeeze (arrowed) the U-loops so that the sides of the U are approximated slightly. Since this adjustment will alter the position of the bow, a further adjustment is then needed (see Figure 4.12).

incisal edge of the tooth to be moved when the appliance is held in position, immediately prior to fully seating it.

The spring should be adjusted by placing the round beak of a pair of Adams' 65 pliers (also known as spring-forming pliers) into the helix that lies closer to the edge of the baseplate, and gently unwinding the helix by pulling the appliance away from the pliers so that the spring moves in a upward and forward direction. The appliance should then be re-inserted into the patient's mouth to check the extent of the activation.

It is important that the free arm of the Z-spring lies parallel to the palatal surface of the tooth to ensure even contact and, hence, even force distribution on the tooth. Point contact on the palatal surface will induce rotational movements. Of course, in teeth that are already rotated, point contact is often all that is possible. However, in these circumstances, the point contact will serve to de-rotate the tooth in question.

The position of the free arm of the Z-spring may be adjusted by placing the round beak of the Adams' 65 pliers in the helix that is closer

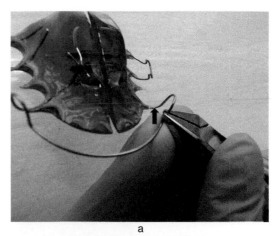

a

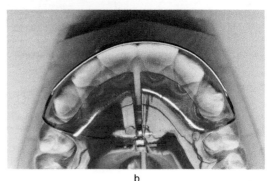

b

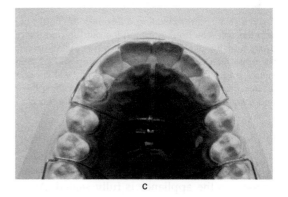

c

Figure 4.12 Tightening the labial bow across the U-loops (see Figure 4.11) results in the anterior section of the labial bow being moved incisally; it must therefore now be pushed gingivally (arrowed; a) so it once more rests in the middle third of the labial surface of the incisors. Before the appliance is fully inserted, the labial bow should lie more or less along the incisal edges (b); so it has to be lifted over the labial surface to sit appropriately (c; and see Figure 4.10).

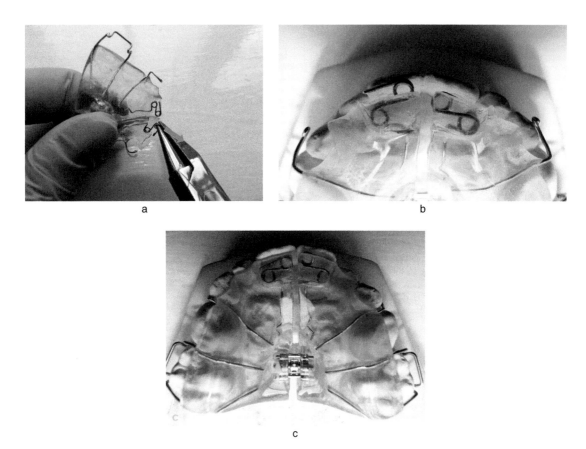

a

b

c

Figure 4.13 (a) Activating a Z-spring: the beaks of the Adams' 65 pliers (also known as spring-forming pliers) grip the coil, one beak gripping the outside and the other the inside the coil. The appliance is then firmly pulled away from the pliers so that the spring is pulled *up* and *away and forward* (arrowed) from the baseplate. Before the appliance is fully inserted, the spring should then lie as shown (b), with the active Z-spring resting at the incisal edge. Once seated (c), the spring will be compressed behind the tooth and will rest approximately in the middle of the palatal surface of the tooth. If the activation only moves the spring forward, rather than up and away from the appliance, then it will lie too close to the incisal edge and will not seat properly.

to the free arm. Gentle finger pressure on the free arm should be used to adjust its position.

Once activated, the Z-spring will be compressed as the appliance is fully seated. As it returns to its original length, it will push the tooth labially, assuming that the height of the posterior capping is adequate to prevent the lower incisors hindering movement. It is this compression that may dislodge the appliance as the Z-spring tries to return to its original length; it tends to slide down the curved palatal surface of the tooth. This is why retention must

be as far anteriorly as possible in appliances with Z-springs and the retention must be really good (Figure 4.13).

T-springs

T-springs are used to move premolar and molar teeth buccally.

As with all active components, the retention of the appliance must be optimised prior to their activation.

T-springs should be positioned with the terminal loop parallel with the palatal bulbosity of the crown of the tooth, and in contact with it.

Activation is achieved by gently raising the T-spring away from the baseplate. The T-spring should now lie more occlusal than the maximum bulbosity of the crown when the appliance is being held in position, immediately before it is fully seated. When fully seated, the T-spring will be compressed back against the maximum bulbosity of the tooth and, as it returns to its uncompressed length, it will push the tooth buccally (Figure 4.14).

As the tooth moves buccally, the length of the T-spring will need to be increased so that it remains in contact with the tooth. This is achieved by releasing some of the wire contained in the 'reservoir' by flattening the loop (Figure 4.15).

Palatal finger springs

Palatal finger springs are used to move teeth mesially and distally around the arch. After checking the seating of the appliance and optimising the retention, the position of the finger spring on the tooth should be checked. The free end of the spring should lie just incisal to the gingival margin of the tooth and, as it emerges from the baseplate, it should curve around the mesial (or distal) aspect of the tooth, in contact with the tooth surface, and finish in a small loop approximately one-third of the distance across the labial surface, still lying just incisal to the gingival margin.

As a general rule, the correct amount of force will be delivered to any given tooth if the spring is activated by one-third of the width of that tooth. The width of the tooth should be measured and with a wax stick, a mark should be made on the baseplate that is one-third of the width of the tooth away from the passive position of the spring in the direction of the desired movement. There are two ways of activating these springs:

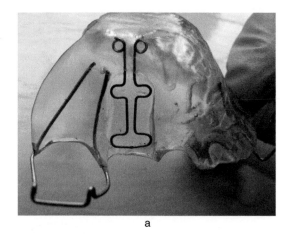

a

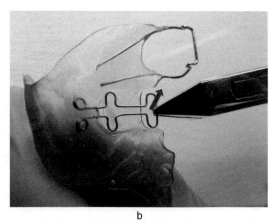

b

Figure 4.14   (a) T-spring; (b) initial activation using spring-forming pliers to pull the free end of the spring *up* and *away* from the baseplate as well as *forward* as shown (arrowed). Future activations require the release of more wire and this is achieved using the reservoir loop (see Figure 4.15).

- The spring-forming pliers grip the wire just in front of the coil (which avoids work hardening the coil), but within the area defined by the guard wire, and the spring is then pushed in the direction in which the tooth is to move (Figure 4.16).
- The round beak of the spring-forming pliers can be placed in the helix of the spring and finger pressure applied to the free arm. It is then adjusted until its new position corresponds to the wax mark on the baseplate.

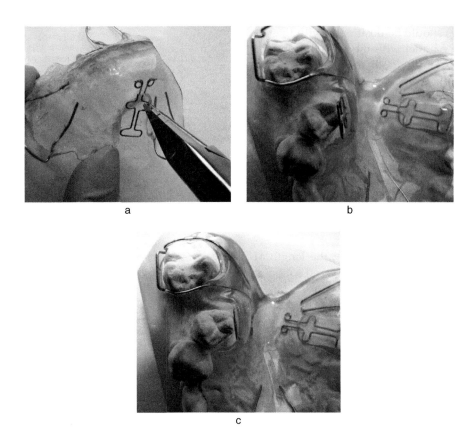

a

b

c

Figure 4.15 Activating the T-spring using the reservoir loops requires the square beak of the spring-forming pliers to be placed inside the reservoir loop and squeezing as shown (a). Since the base of the T-spring is fixed in acrylic, this means the free edge must extend as shown (b). This results in the T-spring resting higher up on the palatal cusp as shown prior to full seating (b). Once fully seated, the spring is compressed against the palatal cusp and is thus active (c).

When the appliance is held in the patient's mouth, immediately before it is fully seated, the spring should now be positioned below the incisal edge/occlusal surface of the tooth, one-third of the tooth width from its original position. Fully seating the appliance will activate the spring by pushing it back to its original passive position. The free arm of the spring will slowly return to its new passive position and, as it does so, it will push the tooth along with it.

After activation, it is important to check that the wire does not impinge on the gingivae or the free end irritate the mucosa of the upper lip.

It is also vitally important that the spring automatically lies in its correct position with no possibility that the patient could insert the appliance with the spring lying against the opposite (incorrect) side of the tooth. If this can occur, then it is likely that the spring has been over-activated and will require further adjustment (correct adjustment is shown in Figure 4.16).

Buccal canine retractors

These springs are only used in one situation – where a canine that needs to be retracted is

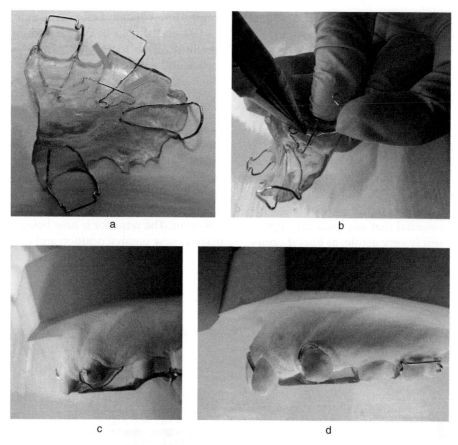

a b

c d

Figure 4.16 (a) Palatal finger spring with box and guard wire (arrowed). (b) To activate it, one method involves placing the spring-forming pliers so that they grip the wire just in front of the coil, but within the area defined by the guard wire, and the spring is then pushed in the direction the tooth is to move. (c) The spring should normally be activated so it lies mesial to the cusp tip (of the canine in this case). If it is being activated on an incisor, then activation is one third of the tooth width (approximately 3 mm). The active palatal finger spring is now seated as shown (d), ensuring that it fits closely against the tooth, around the gingival margin.

buccally displaced and mesially angulated. Correction of upper canine position is more efficiently and more optimally performed using fixed appliances.

The correct positioning of a buccal canine retractor is imperative, not only for the purposes of tooth movement, but because incorrect positioning may cause the patient a significant amount of pain if the helix traumatises the buccal sulcus. The position of the canine retractor should be checked with the circum-oral muscles relaxed, but the patient must also be

asked to talk, laugh, swallow and simulate eating in order to check that the retractor does not impinge on the buccal sulcus during oral functions. Unlike dentures, the appliance will not be dislodged by muscle activity because of the significantly increased retention provided by the Adams' clasps. The fly-over should lie close to, or in contact with, the contact point between the upper premolar teeth. It is also very important to check that the sleeved arm of the retractor does not impinge on the gingivae. The free end of the spring should curve around the mesial aspect of the canine, just incisal to the gingival margin, and should finish in a small loop.

Activation should be by one-third of the width of the tooth, as with palatal finger springs. The same technique should be used, measuring the width of the tooth and marking one-third of this width on the baseplate distal to the passive position of the retractor. The round beak of the Adams' 65 pliers should be placed in the helix and gentle finger pressure applied to the free arm until its new passive position corresponds to the mark on the baseplate. It is essential that any pressure applied to the free arm is very gentle, as buccal canine retractors distort easily and, hence, fit less well. When the appliance is held in the patient's mouth, immediately before it is fully seated, the free end should lie on the occlusal aspect, one-third of the tooth width from the mesial surface and mesial to the cusp tip of the canine. When the appliance is fully seated, the free end should slide down the curved mesial surface of the canine and come to lie with its free end in its original position, curved around the mesial aspect of the tooth, just occlusal to the gingival margins. The position of the helix, the sleeved arm and the free end should all be re-checked after activation to ensure that they are all still in the correct place and no iatrogenic damage can occur. The retractor is now being stretched from its new passive position and as it returns to its passive length it will push the tooth along with it (Figure 4.17).

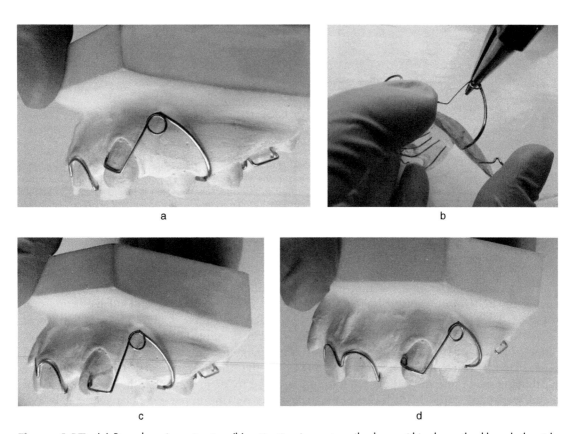

a   b
c   d

Figure 4.17 (a) Buccal canine retractor; (b) activation is most easily done within the coil, although the risk of wire fracture exists due to work hardening; (c) the appropriate amount of activation; (d) the position of the activated spring with the appliance fully inserted.

Labial bows

When labial bows are used as an active component rather than a retentive component, although adjustment is still made at the U-loops, there are some important differences.

As the appliance is being used to retract the incisors, space is required into which these teeth can move. The space is gained by trimming away the acrylic of the baseplate to provide a gap of around 1.5 mm between the palatal surfaces of the incisors and the most anterior aspect of the baseplate. However, it is vitally important that the baseplate is not trimmed so much that it no longer controls the position of the lower incisor teeth as these will over-erupt and prevent the upper incisors from moving palatally. The fit surface of the baseplate should also be chamfered adjacent to the margin that has just been trimmed in order to accommodate the 'bow wave' of palatal mucosa that will appear once the teeth start to move. The gingival tissues take longer to remodel than the bone surrounding the teeth, and whilst they will flatten over a period of time, they do become a little bulky initially as they are pushed from behind by the teeth, hence the necessity to chamfer the baseplate.

Once space has been created, the labial bow is activated in the same manner in which retention is increased; by squeezing the U-loops. The general rule is that the bow should be activated so that it comes to lie just incisal to the incisal edges of the teeth when held in position prior to being fully seated. When the appliance is fully seated, the bow should be positioned in the middle third of the crown. When it is in this position, it will be stretched from its passive position and will move the teeth palatally as it returns to its passive position (Figure 4.12).

Expansion screws

These require the full co-operation of the patient, because their activation requires the turning of a key in the screw on a weekly or twice-weekly basis.

All appliances that contain expansion screws should have an arrow marked on the baseplate to indicate the direction in which the screw should be turned by the key. This arrow is routinely embedded in any screw appliance by the technician and will be distinctively coloured to stand out from the background baseplate colour. The expansion screw contains four holes, two of which are visible at any one time. The key should be inserted into the hole that is closer to the back of the arrow and should then be turned in the direction of the arrow until it can move no further (Figure 4.18). The key should then be removed and the appliance re-inserted into the patient's mouth. In reality, the key will have turned the screw by a one-quarter turn. This activation will have opened up the split in the baseplate by 0.25 mm, which is the average width of the periodontal ligament. This is why only a single activation (a one-quarter turn) should be completed at any one time. If the screw is activated by more than this, the blood vessels in the periodontal ligament run the risk of being occluded, leading to hyalinisation and undermining resorption.

It is imperative that both the patient and the parent are shown how to activate the expansion screw and that the importance of this to the success of treatment is emphasised. Many patients actually like the fact that they are actively involved in their treatment and co-operation is rarely a problem given appropriate communication from the clinician. The key should be placed in the appliance container for safe-keeping.

Elastics

These require good patient co-operation and much more manual dexterity from the patient/parent/guardian than the expansion screw.

These days, elastics are seldom used with URAs, apart from the extrusion of a tooth (incisor) during the mixed dentition stage. However, they are very effective for this as long as the patient is able to change the elastic band on a daily basis. Significant encouragement must be given to the patient, but as the appearance

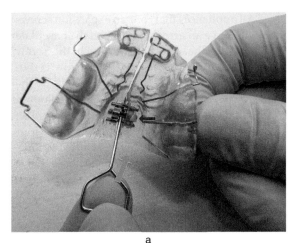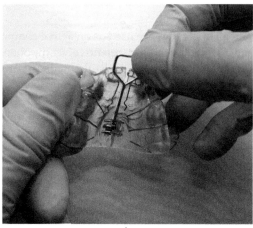

a   b

Figure 4.18 Turning the screw in an upper removable appliance. (a) The key is inserted into the screw hole toward the rear of the appliance; it will be turned in the direction of the yellow arrow embedded in the appliance baseplate. The yellow arrow (embedded in the baseplate) is highlighted by the dark blue arrow in this illustration. Whenever a screw appliance is made, the technician will routinely embed an arrow in the appliance baseplate, indicating the direction in which to turn the key. (b) The key is then turned *forward* in the direction this arrow until it cannot be turned any further. This results in a one-quarter turn of the screw, in the direction of the arrow.

of an upper incisor that requires extrusion is often unsightly, the patient is often very determined to do whatever is necessary to improve the appearance.

Instructing the patient/parent/guardian on insertion and removal of the appliance

Once you think that you have completed adjusting the appliance in terms of fit, retention and activation, it is important to check with the patient whether any component is uncomfortable or is digging in, although they should accept that the appliance will feel very strange at first. Once this has been checked, it is time to demonstrate to the patient how to put the appliance in and take it out.

It is essential that the patient's ability to insert and remove the appliance is confirmed prior to them leaving the surgery. Knowing that they are able to deal with the appliance by themselves gives the patient confidence, and the encouragement and praise that can be given to the patient when they show they are able to insert and remove the appliance is very valuable in ensuring success of the treatment.

The patient should be sitting upright when the insertion and removal of an appliance is demonstrated.

- Demonstrate appliance removal first, as this is easier for the patient.
- Place the appliance in the patient's mouth and provide them with a mirror so that they can see what you are doing in their mouth.
- Show the patient how to remove the appliance, giving clear verbal instructions as you demonstrate this.
- It is very important to inform the patient that firm finger pressure is required on the clasps around the back teeth. Patients are often surprised how much force is required to dislodge a retentive appliance.
- It is also very important that appliances are not removed by initially pushing on the anterior retentive components or any active components. This may distort these components and potentially cause the incorrect amount or direction of force to be placed on the teeth.

- Once the appliance has been removed, show it to the patient and indicate which components are to fit around which teeth, e.g. 'these clasps go around your back teeth'.
- Demonstrate and talk though the key steps to inserting the appliance, with the patient watching in the mirror.
- Advise the patient to position the appliance in their mouth, check that the springs are in the correct place, and then push up firmly on the acrylic until a click is heard and the appliance is in place.

Now the patient needs to demonstrate to you that they can remove and insert the appliance:

- Ask your nurse to hold the mirror for the patient, leaving your gloved hands free to help the patient.
- Many patients will try to remove the appliance by pulling down on the first piece of wire-work they see, so it is important to remind them (in lay terms) to place their fingers over the bridges of the clasps on the molars and pull down hard.
- At this stage, the appliance will be covered with copious amounts of saliva, which causes most patients to say 'ugh'. It is essential to be ready with tissues and lots of positive encouragement – the 'dribbling' only lasts 1–2 hours.
- When the excess saliva has been removed, ask the patient to put the appliance back in their mouth, offering verbal encouragement and reminders as necessary.
- Always demonstrate again the correct position of the springs before the appliance is fully seated.
- Once the appliance is in place, check that it has been inserted correctly and give the patient lots of praise.

Ask the patient and the parent/guardian if they are confident in being able to remove and insert the appliance at home by themselves. The majority of patients are able to manage the insertion and removal of appliances very well

and only a very few will need to repeat the process with you watching.

Instructions and advice to the patient and parent/guardian

There are a number of instructions and pieces of advice that must be imparted to the patient and parent/guardian; most importantly, the dentist must be very enthusiastic in 'selling' the appliance to the patient and parent. A lukewarm reaction by the clinician is guaranteed to make the patient less enthusiastic about wearing it and the parent less likely to encourage/enforce wear at home.

When should the appliance be worn?

With the exception of retainers (which will be dealt with in separate chapters) all appliances, both active and passive, should be worn on a full-time basis, ideally 24 hours per day, including in bed, whilst eating and at school. However, having said that, there are obviously occasions when the appliance must be removed for dental health reasons. These are:

- When the patient is undertaking oral hygiene measures
- After every meal in order that food debris may be rinsed off the appliance
- During contact sports
- When swimming.

When the appliance is not being worn, it should be kept safe in a plastic container, either a specifically provided appliance container or a small food container.

How should the appliance be cared for?

The appliance should be removed after every meal and rinsed under a tap to remove food debris. It should be cleaned using a toothbrush and toothpaste, preferably over a bowl of water to prevent damage from the appliance being dropped into a porcelain washbasin. This should be carried out at least three times a day i.e. after each meal.

Should the appliance be worn when eating?

The answer to this question is always an unqualified 'Yes'. The reason for this is that if the patient removes the appliance when eating, then the occlusal forces are at their most frequent and forceful, and can return a tooth toward its original position. Therefore, all the good the appliance has done is rapidly lost due to relapse. This not only delays treatment, but may damage the tooth-supporting structures due to 'jiggling' forces caused by the tooth being pushed to and fro by the appliance and the occlusion. This should be explained to the patient and parent. Furthermore, for some appliances, wear during meal times will help the active components be at their most effective. Of course, on top of these factors, if a patient takes the appliance out at meal times, there is a risk they will forget to re-insert it or even lose it, which compounds the problems still further. Therefore, it is essential to advise that whilst eating with the appliance in the mouth will be difficult initially, it is a good idea to eat soft food until they get used to eating with the appliance in place.

Will the appliance hurt?

With active appliances, the teeth will be uncomfortable as they start to move. The force applied to the teeth by the appliance will take approximately 6 hours to induce the cellular changes necessary to cause bone resorption and deposition to commense. As this process occurs via a sterile inflammation, pain-inducing substances, e.g. prostaglandins, are produced, causing tooth discomfort. The discomfort begins 4–6 hours after an active appliance has been first fitted and after each time it has been reacti-

vated. The discomfort lasts between 3 and 7 days and the amount of discomfort felt varies between patients depending on a number of appliance/tooth-related factors, but also the patient's pain tolerance. Advice should be given to the patient and, especially, the parent/guardian that, if the teeth do feel very uncomfortable, whatever analgesia the patient would normally take to cure a headache should be taken. It is important to stress that the patient does not exceed the maximum safe dose for the particular analgesic.

The wire or acrylic components of the appliance may cause discomfort by rubbing on the oral mucosa. This will only last for 10–14 days, until the oral mucosa has generated a thicker layer of keratin to protect it from the appliance.

Oral hygiene measures

Even if the patient's oral hygiene is very good, which, of course, it should be prior to fitting an appliance, it is necessary to re-inforce the importance of good oral hygiene and good dietary control at every appointment. Removal of the appliance for tooth-brushing must be emphasised. Although it may seem obvious, it is surprising how many patients attempt to brush their teeth with their appliances *in situ*!

Fluoride mouthwash

The use of a fluoride mouthwash at a 0.05% concentration on a daily basis is the one measure that has been shown to reduce the incidence of demineralisation during orthodontic treatment with fixed appliances, as concluded in a Cochrane systematic review, (Benson *et al.*, 2004). However, as a removable appliance is also a plaque-retention factor, patients who are wearing removable appliances should also be advised to use a daily mouthwash that contains fluoride at a concentration of 0.05%. Some fluoride mouthwashes contain enough fluoride within a bottle to be toxic to a small child, but the bottles do not come with child-proof tops. Therefore, it is essential to warn all parents that the mouthwash should be kept in a cupboard that is out of reach of young siblings or young visitors.

What should the patient do if the appliance breaks or is loose or digs in?

The patient and carer should be advised that should the appliance break or become too loose, then they should contact the surgery urgently for advice. The clinician should therefore have arrangements in place to deal with such problems urgently – within 1 or 2 days – since otherwise, if the appliance cannot be worn properly, it will not work and/or any progress that has been made will be lost through relapse. Such problems will require the patient to call in for repair or adjustment as needed. Obviously, adjustments such as tightening a loose appliance can be quickly undertaken, but more time will be required if the appliance needs to be repaired; the sooner the patient can attend, the sooner the problem can start to be addressed.

If a repair is needed, this will usually require access to laboratory facilities and the patient will need to make a further visit once the repair is ready to be fitted. If a whole new clasp or spring is needed, then an impression with the appliance in place will be needed.

In some situations, it may be possible for the fractured ends of a clasp (or bow) to be soldered together, but this can only be considered where the ends are at least 2 mm from the acrylic baseplate. This is not however, usually possible for springs.

The above advice should be provided verbally to the patient and the parent after the appliance has been fitted, and whilst they are still in the surgery. Adequate time should be allowed at the end of each fitting appointment so that the instructions on wear may be provided in an unhurried manner and the patient and parent are given plenty of opportunity to ask questions.

It can therefore be seen that it is good practice to provide the patient with a Patient Information Leaflet (PIL) listing all the advice that has been provided verbally; this can act as a first point of reference if the patient is unsure of anything once they have left the surgery. This PIL should also contain a telephone number that the patient may phone in order to ask for advice if they have any concerns.

Finally, before the patient and parent/guardian leave the surgery, a follow-up appointment should be arranged in 4–6 weeks at a time that is mutually convenient for all concerned.

Reference

Benson PE, Parkin N, Millett DT, Dyer F, Vine S, Shah A (2004) Fluorides for the prevention of white spots on teeth during fixed brace treatment. *Cochrane Database of Systematic Reviews* Issue 3: CD003809.

Follow-up Appointments: What to Check and Why

5

It is obvious to all that follow-up appointments are an essential part of orthodontic treatment and these fulfil a number of roles, not only to check on the amount of tooth movement. They should also be used to check on oral hygiene and patient co-operation, and to provide praise and encouragement, as appropriate.

Learning outcomes

At the end of this chapter you should have knowledge and understanding of:

- What to monitor at regular follow-up appointments
- How to spot when something is going wrong
- The necessary adjustments to removable appliances
- How to manage the end of treatment and retention
- What not to treat
- How/when to refer

Appointment frequency

Once the removable appliance has been fitted and activated, it will be necessary to review the patient's progress at regular intervals; every 4–6 weeks. This time interval is ideal because it allows plenty of time for the appliance to work and for the cellular processes involved to settle once more. If any shorter than this, the appliance may not have fully achieved the tooth movement it should do. Furthermore, it may also predispose to root resorption if the appliance is re-activated too frequently. If any longer than 4–6 weeks, treatment progress may be delayed since the appliance will become passive and lie idle, and the period of time for which the appliance needs to be worn will be lengthened. Of course, the patient and parents/guardian should be fully aware that regular appointments will be required as part of the informed consent process and before the appliance is fitted.

Orthodontic Retainers and Removable Appliances: Principles of Design and Use, First Edition.
Friedy Luther and Zararna Nelson-Moon.
© 2013 Friedy Luther and Zararna Nelson-Moon. Published 2013 by Blackwell Publishing Ltd.

Tooth movement, trouble-shooting and adjustments to the appliance will be covered for each type of tooth movement.

What to monitor

There are a number of key markers that must be observed at each follow-up appointment:

- Whether the patient is wearing the appliance as requested
- Oral hygiene
- The maintenance of the appliance
- Tooth movement, both wanted and unwanted.

Obviously, there is some overlap between these areas, but performing the examination of the patient in a systematic and logical manner will ensure that nothing is forgotten.

Is the patient wearing the appliance, and how?

Perhaps the first and most telling sign that a patient has not been wearing their appliance as requested is that they still have a pronounced lisp on speaking with the appliance in place. If an appliance is being worn appropriately, speech, in the vast majority of individuals, will return to normal within 1–2 days of having the appliance fitted as the tongue adapts to the thickness of the acrylic baseplate over the palate.

If the patient has worn the appliance, they will be able to insert and remove the appliance with ease, without the need for a mirror or any help. It is likely that a patient who demonstrates difficulty when attempting to remove or insert the appliance has not been wearing the appliance as requested.

Also, an appliance that has been worn becomes loose as the wire-work of the retentive components deflects on removal and insertion and, eventually, plastically deforms. An appliance that has not been worn remains 'tight' and requires some effort to remove.

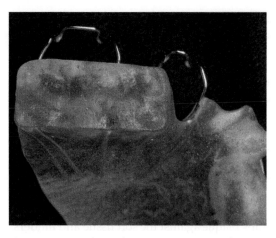

Figure 5.1 URA with posterior capping showing wear.

An appliance that has been worn shows signs of wear: either tooth marks on the acrylic (if biteplanes/capping have been included in the design) or tarnishing of the metal components. An appliance that still has completely clear acrylic with no signs of occlusal wear (and whose wire-work is still very shiny) has not been worn appropriately (Figure 5.1).

It is necessary to check that the appliance is being inserted correctly by the patient and that any active components, especially palatal finger springs, are being placed on the correct side of each tooth.

If the appliance does not seat as well as it did at the fitting appointment, this is an indication that the appliance has been left out of the mouth for at least a few days, allowing teeth to move independently. This is especially the case in patients whose permanent teeth are erupting or whose teeth have been removed, allowing adjacent teeth to tip into the extraction sites.

Oral hygiene

The standard of oral hygiene often deteriorates when an orthodontic appliance is first fitted, even though the removable appliance should be taken out during oral hygiene measures.

Patients will often brush their teeth well immediately before their dental/orthodontic appointment and *so it is important to check the health of the gingivae and the appliance hygiene*, as well as the cleanliness of the teeth.

Gingivitis may be hidden. It is commonly occurs on the *palatal/lingual* gingival margins when wearing a removable appliance, especially if the appliance is not removed each time the teeth are brushed and/or oral hygiene measures are inadequate.

Also, the palatal/lingual gingival margins are covered by the removable appliance, which traps plaque against the soft tissue and hinders the anti-bacterial properties of the saliva from reaching the gingival margins. This also leads to more plaque build up on the palatal/lingual surfaces of the teeth, compounding the problem (Figure 5.2).

Poor *appliance* hygiene can be a significant problem, especially in younger patients. Plaque left on the fit surface of the acrylic baseplate not only exacerbates the gingivitis, but can cause a denture-stomatitis type of reaction to the palatal mucosa. This is due to the presence of candida species being held in contact with the palatal mucosa by the fit surface of the appliance (Figure 5.3).

Initial treatment of this condition should concentrate on improving the appliance hygiene, ensuring that the appliance is thoroughly cleaned three times per day with the patient's toothbrush and toothpaste. With denture stomatitis from wearing a denture, the patient can be advised to leave the appliance out at night. In contrast, this cannot be advised for patients who are wearing an active orthodontic appliance, as if the appliance is left out overnight and therefore for 8-hour periods, the teeth will start moving back (relapsing) and prevent the appliance from seating properly. If the stomatitis does not resolve with improved oral hygiene, then it may be necessary to prescribe a course of topical miconazole (an anti-fungal), which should be placed on the fit surface of the appliance.

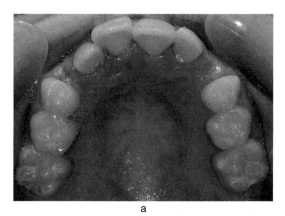

a

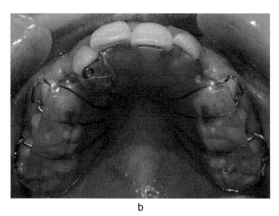

b

Figure 5.2 Oral health can easily deteriorate under a URA (a). Note the gingival inflammation around all the palatal gingival margins and buccally where there is also staining. The appliance associated with the poor oral hygiene is shown (b).

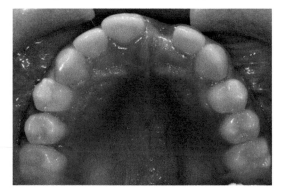

Figure 5.3 A denture-stomatitis type of reaction affecting the palatal mucosa is caused by poor *appliance* hygiene.

Maintenance of the appliance

All appliances that are being worn appropriately become loose between review appointments, as described above. Therefore, at each review appointment, it will generally be necessary to increase the retention of the appliance, as detailed in Chapter 4. Obviously, any active components will require re-activation.

However, it is also important to check thoroughly the overall status of the appliance to ensure that the wire-work has not fractured and that no acrylic has been lost. This usually occurs on anterior biteplanes or posterior capping, due to the occlusal forces, but may occur anywhere on the baseplate. It is often possible just to remove any sharp edges from the acrylic, but if a large piece has fractured off an anterior biteplane or posterior capping, it may be that the appliance is no longer controlling the eruption/position of certain teeth. If this is the case, then the appliance will need to be repaired, either at the chairside using cold-cure acrylic or by a laboratory.

Any damage to the wire-work should also be assessed. Damage can occur in the form of distortion or fracture. Distortion is usually caused by the patient removing the appliance in the wrong way, e.g. pulling down on the labial bow, rather than applying a downward force on the clasps. Other reasons for distortion include: inserting the appliance with the springs in the wrong position or the appliance being sat on!

Fracture of the wire-work occurs where the metal has been work hardened due to repeated reactivation, e.g. by the arrowheads of the Adams' clasps (Figure 5.4) or the U-loops of a labial bow, or because of repeated flexion of the wire due to occlusal trauma, e.g. the fly-overs of retentive components such as clasps and labial bows.

Whenever an active, removable appliance needs to be removed to be repaired, you must remember that any teeth that have been moved will start to drift back toward their starting position within hours of the appliance being

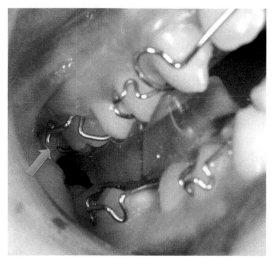

Figure 5.4 A fractured Adams' clasp (arrowed).

taken out. Therefore, if the appliance can be repaired to a satisfactory standard at the chairside, or there is a laboratory on site, then this is preferable to having to leave the patient without the appliance for a few days. If the appliance does need to be sent to a laboratory, remember to de-activate the active components a little before re-fitting the appliance once it returns from the laboratory.

Tooth movement, both wanted and unwanted, and adjustments

In order to be certain that tooth movement has occurred appropriately, it is essential to compare the patient's dentition *at each visit* with the pre-treatment study models and to note details of the:

- Overjet
- Overbite
- Canine and molar relationships
- Size of any spaces (this includes measuring spaces and checking they are not closing during space maintenance)/open bites
- Transverse relationships – depending on what movement you are trying to achieve.

However, it is very important to be aware of the direction in which unwanted tooth movements may occur, e.g. due to loss of anchorage, and to check thoroughly at each visit that unwanted movements are not occurring, especially if there does not appear to be any movement of the tooth/teeth that you are attempting to move with the appliance.

If such measurements are not taken regularly, assessing treatment progress becomes impossible as any developing problems will be missed; it is not appropriate to rely on one's memory.

Adjustments at follow-up appointments

Retentive components almost always need to be adjusted to increase the retention of the appliance and, obviously, active components, e.g. springs, will need to be re-activated. Always adjust the retention before reactivating the springs. However, there are other specific adjustments that are required depending on exactly what type of tooth movement you are trying to achieve.

Expansion

What to check

Improvement in, or correction of, the posterior crossbite is obviously a good indication that expansion has occurred. Likewise, no change in the occlusion indicates that the appliance is not being worn. However, since it is likely to take several months to correct a posterior crossbite, one needs to be able to assess whether improvements are taking place from visit to visit. This can be done by measuring the width between two obvious landmarks at each review visit. For example, the inter-molar width can be measured between the mesio-buccal cusp tips using dividers and a ruler (Figure 5.5) or Vernier divider.

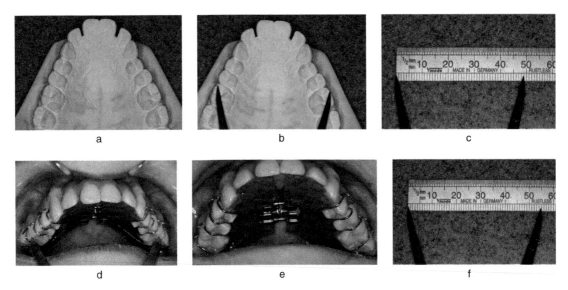

Figure 5.5 When the inter-molar width is to be expanded, the amount of expansion needs to be measured at each visit. Dividers and a ruler can be used as shown here. The upper model (a) is initially measured using clear landmarks such as U6 mesio-buccal cusp widths (b). This width is measured on the ruler (c) and noted. This measurement can then be repeated at future visits (d), each width being recorded in the patient's records. Here, expansion has progressed (e), from 49 mm (c) to 55 mm (f).

Trouble-shooting

The following need to be checked when all the indications are that the patient has been wearing the appliance, yet there has been minimal improvement in transverse discrepancy since the patient was last reviewed:

- That the patient is turning the expansion screw in the right direction, by the correct amount and the requested number of times per week. It is possible to check all of these by turning the screw backward yourself and counting how many turns you are able to make, e.g. if you have asked the patient to turn the screw *twice* per week and it is *6 weeks* since you last saw them, then you should be able to turn the screw backward by *12 ¼ turns*. If you cannot, then you should question the patient and/or parent/guardian regarding the activation. It is also advisable to ask the patient and/or parent/guardian to demonstrate to you how they are turning the screw. You may be surprised. Also, the split in the baseplate should have opened by a set number of millimetres, calculated by multiplying the number of ¼ turns of the screw made by the patient by 0.25 mm (the amount of expansion per ¼ turn). So, in the example above, the split in the baseplate should have widened by 3 mm.
- Whether the lower arch has expanded as well. If posterior capping was included in the design to disengage the occlusion, then this should not happen. However, it is very straightforward to check whether this has happened by measuring between two clearly defined points on the study models, e.g. the mesio-buccal cusps of the lower first permanent molar teeth, and comparing this with the same measurement taken in the patient's mouth. The measurement should be the same in the mouth as on the study models. If the measurement in the mouth is greater than on the study models, then some expansion of the lower arch has occurred and you

need to check for occlusal interferences in the transverse dimension.

- Whether the appliance has been left out for any reason and some relapse of the expansion has already occurred. This will be very apparent as the appliance will not fit properly because it will be wider than the dentition. The reason that the patient has stopped wearing the appliance needs to be investigated thoroughly, as, if the reason persists, compliance with wear will continue to be poor.
- It is unlikely that anchorage will be lost in expansion cases as anchorage is usually reciprocal.

Next stage

If the expansion is going well and the patient is compliant, then all that is necessary at this stage is to determine whether further expansion is required to fully correct the crossbite. It is always useful to overcorrect if possible, because a little bit of relapse of the tooth movement is to be expected. If further expansion is required, then the patient should be asked to continue turning the screw once or twice per week.

Moving teeth around the arch

When teeth are being moved around the arch, they are usually being tipped, either mesially or distally, into a space, so that as the teeth move, the space relocates. However, it is very easy to lose anchorage when teeth are being moved in this way, especially if more than one tooth is being moved at any one time in the same direction. Therefore, it is imperative that the position of the anchor teeth and overjet are also checked at every review appointment.

What to check

Good indications that the teeth are being moved in the appropriate manner are:

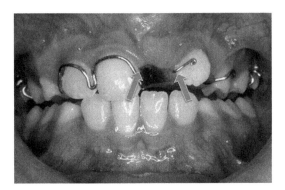

Figure 5.6 In this case, a URA is being used to retract UL2 out of the UL1 space. In order to assess progress, the space between UR1 and UL2 (arrowed) should be measured with dividers at each visit.

- The teeth to be moved are in a different position in the mouth from on the study models.
- Measure the space you are moving the tooth into. Depending on what is planned, of course the space should get smaller or larger at each visit. Again this movement can be measured with dividers and a ruler or Vernier dividers. Figure 5.6 shows a space being opened and demonstrates the gap to be measured:
- There is now more space apparent behind the tooth
- There is an increased tip on the tooth, in the direction of movement
- There has been no movement of any of the other teeth that are in contact with the appliance (the anchor teeth).

All of the above indicate that the appliance has been worn well by the patient and that the amount of force delivered by the active component is appropriate.

Trouble-shooting

However, if the above points are not evident and you are certain that the patient's compliance with your instructions has been good, then you need to consider if the force applied by the active component has been too large? If so, the tooth to be moved is likely still to have moved, albeit in a step-wise rather than continuous manner. This is due to the occurrence of hyalinisation in the periodontal ligament followed by undermining resorption of the alveolar bone. This may take 10–14 days. During this time period the tooth is prevented from moving, but the force from the active component continues to be dissipated to all the other teeth in contact with the appliance (the anchor teeth), but in the opposite direction. If the threshold force level required for tooth movement is exceeded, then the anchor teeth will move.

Example: Consider the case of a removable appliance to distalise UR2, UL1 and UL2 to recreate space to allow the eruption of UR1 (design shown in Figure 3.4). If the combined force placed on these teeth exceeds the force threshold for movement on the anchor teeth (because either excessive force levels are being used or too many teeth are being moved at the same time), then the following effects will be seen:

- The space between UR2 and UL1 will have increased. *If this is the only thing that is checked, then this can give the erroneous impression that the treatment is going well.*
- The space distal to UR2 and UL2 will have decreased significantly.
- The overjet will have increased.
- The molar relationship will have become more Class II.

These effects are all due to loss of anchorage, with the anchor teeth moving in the opposite direction to the teeth to be moved. Once anchorage has been lost, rescuing the situation is very difficult.

Next stage

Assuming tooth movement is progressing as planned, then the following adjustments need to be made to the appliance:

- Adjust the retention as necessary, ensuring that the arrowheads of the clasps do not impinge on the gingivae.
- Check that there is no hindrance to further tooth movement in the form of acrylic collets, wire-work or the occlusion.
- Check that palatal finger springs can still move freely and that there has been no distortion.
- Re-activate the springs by the required amount.
- Check that the springs are still adapted around the tooth appropriately.
- As the last check, ensure that the appliance is comfortable for the patient and that the patient can still remove and insert the appliance appropriately.

You may wish to refer to Chapter 4 for a recap on activation and adjustment of clasps and springs.

If anchorage has been lost, resulting in a change in molar relationship and an increase in overjet, then you will need to ask for the advice/services of a specialist orthodontist (see later). If things are not going well, it is best to seek advice early. Do not just leave things to get worse.

Moving teeth labially

What to check

Anterior crossbites are often treated very quickly (in 3 or 4 months) in a compliant patient and when the treatment has been planned appropriately. This is because appliances of the sort shown in Chapter 2 (see Figure 2.2) automatically eliminate the mandibular displacement by disengaging the occlusion, leaving the teeth to move only a small distance for a positive overjet to be achieved. Teeth that have been held in a retroclined position due to the crossbite often have some spontaneous improvement in position – purely as an effect of disengaging the occlusion.

- There should no longer be a mandibular displacement, even when the appliance is not in place, as the posterior capping on the URA will have helped to de-programme the muscles of mastication if the URA has been worn as prescribed.
- There should be an edge-to-edge incisor relationship or better.
- Check that there is still enough occlusal clearance to allow further labial movement of the relevant teeth.

Trouble-shooting

If there has been little progress in eliminating the crossbite, despite all the indications that the patient is compliant with instructions, it needs to be checked if the incisors have 'erupted' to such an extent that there is no longer an anterior open bite with the appliance in place. In an actively growing individual, one would expect the incisors to erupt further when the occlusion is disengaged using posterior capping. Of course, this is very beneficial because it aids end-of-treatment retention by increasing the overbite. However, a significant and rapid overbite increase is likely to prevent labial movement of the upper teeth. If the upper incisors engage the lingual of the lower incisors, movement of the upper teeth is possible, but the crossbite will not be corrected because the lower incisors become proclined as the upper incisors are pushed against the lingual aspect. This stresses the periodontium of the lower labial segment (LLS), causing gingival recession. In this situation, more acrylic will need to be added to the posterior capping to free up the occlusion.

Next stage

- Adjust the retention as necessary, ensuring that the arrowheads of the clasps do not impinge on the gingivae.
- Check that there is no hindrance to further tooth movement in the form of wire-work or the occlusion.

- Re-activate the Z-springs by the required amount.
- Check that the springs are still adapted to the palatal surface of the tooth.
- Ensure that the appliance is comfortable for the patient and that the patient can still remove and insert it appropriately.

Reduction of overbite

What to check

If the appliance is being worn appropriately, the overbite will reduce, even in an adult patient, although it will take longer. In a child or adolescent patient, the overbite is reduced very rapidly. In a compliant patient, one can see some overbite reduction occurring in just a few days (Figure 5.7). Evidence of overbite reduction includes:

- The overbite is no longer complete to tooth (or mucosa) when the appliance is out of the mouth.
- There is less separation of the buccal teeth when the appliance is in the mouth than when it was first fitted.

Trouble-shooting

Assuming the anterior biteplane is appropriately active, the only reason for an overbite not reducing in a growing patient is that the patient is not compliant.

Next stage

Because the tooth movement is very rapid, it is necessary to check at each visit that the posterior teeth are not in contact when the appliance is in place. Once the posterior teeth are in

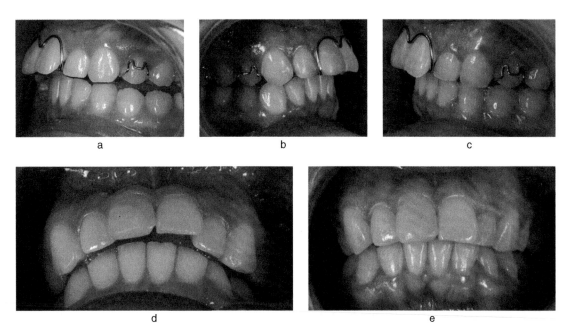

a   b   c

d   e

Figure 5.7   This is the same patient as shown in Figure 4.3. When the flat anterior biteplane (FABP) is first fitted, the active FABP separates the buccal teeth by approximately 2 mm (a). After 3 months' wear of the FABP, note that the buccal teeth are now in contact (b and c). Conversely, the lower incisors no longer occlude with the palatal gingival margins of the upper incisors (d) and the overbite can be seen to be reduced when the patient occludes without the appliance in place (e).

contact, no more overbite reduction can occur. Therefore, if more overbite reduction is required, acrylic should be added to the anterior biteplane (and adjusted as described previously) so that the posterior teeth are out of occlusion once more.

Reducing an overjet

What to check

As stated in and described in detail in Chapter 4, removable appliances should nowadays only be used to reduce an overjet in a very specific situation: where the overjet is only slightly increased and where the upper incisors are only very mildly proclined and spaced. These circumstances may allow the upper incisors to be retroclined, resulting in the overjet being reduced, but without compromising aesthetics. Therefore, first check whether the overjet has reduced (use a ruler) and whether any spaces are reducing in size. However, as this movement also stresses the anchorage, it is absolutely essential that the molar relationship, as well as the overjet reduction, is checked at each visit. If the molar relationship is becoming more Class II, then this is an indication that anchorage is being lost.

Trouble-shooting

If the activation on the labial bow is appropriate, there are still a number of reasons why the overjet may not reduce and/or the anchorage may be lost. These are:

- The upper incisors are being prevented from moving palatally by the acrylic of the baseplate.
- The upper incisors are being prevented from moving palatally by the lower incisors, i.e. a deep and/or complete overbite.

Next stage

It is important to trim the acrylic away from the palatal surfaces of the upper incisors at every visit, but equally important not to trim the acrylic back so far that the lower incisors are no longer biting on the acrylic. If the biteplane is trimmed back too much, it will allow the lower incisors to over-erupt, increasing the overbite and so preventing upper incisor movement.

It is also important to ensure that the upper incisors are not becoming too retroclined. If this is the case, then a referral to a specialist will be necessary. However, this suggests the case was inappropriately assessed in the first place.

Extrusion of incisors

If the patient is compliant and the tooth is not ankylosed, extrusion may occur quite rapidly. However, it is not ideal for the tooth to come down too quickly (due to the risk of compromising the vascular supply to the pulp), but often there is some spontaneous eruption as well.

What to check

At each visit, the movement of the tooth should be measured against a clearly defined object, e.g. the incisal edge of the adjacent incisor, and the measurement recorded in the clinical notes. The degree to which the incisor is being pulled palatally by the direction of pull of the elastic should also be monitored, especially in relation to whether the patient is developing an edge-to-edge bite, or even a frank crossbite, on this tooth.

Trouble-shooting

If the tooth is not moving, then it is important to assess the following:

- Is the tooth ankylosed? Sometimes, it is not possible to tell whether or not a tooth is ankylosed before trying to move it. If the patient is compliant and the mechanics are correct, then a lack of movement indicates

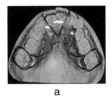
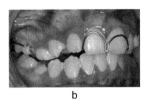
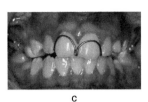
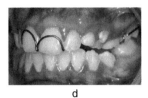

a   b   c   d

Figure 5.8 An example of a space maintainer on its working model (a) and in the mouth (b–d). UR4 and UL4 are to be removed (together with ULC and ULD) to enable the eruption of the permanent upper canines into the line of the arch. In this example, prevention of drift of the teeth is reliant on the acrylic colleting. A more reliable method would involve the addition of wire stops (see Figure 3.17).

ankylosis, especially in a tooth that has been intruded due to trauma. It may be possible to detect the ankylosis by the 'cracked cup' sound that an ankylosed tooth makes when tapped with a metal instrument, e.g. the handle of an oral examination mirror – very different from the 'dull-thud' sound of a tooth that is not ankylosed. Intrusion of adjacent teeth is a more definitive indicator of ankylosis.

- The amount of activation on the elastic band. Although it will be necessary to start extrusive traction with a large elastic band that can stretch far enough to only deliver a very light force to the tooth (maximum 50 g), it is necessary to check at each visit that there is still enough activation with that size of elastic band. If there is little or no activation, then it will be necessary to change to a smaller elastic band in order to generate the required force levels.

Next stage

At each appointment you will need to measure the position of the tooth that is being moved and record this in the notes, as detailed above. Ensure that the acrylic baseplate is not hindering the extrusive movement, but also ensure that it is kept in contact with the palatal surface of the incisor. This is to prevent it moving palatally. Change the size of elastics as necessary and check that the patient can still apply a smaller size of elastic and that they are chang-

ing the elastic every day (or replacing it straightaway should it snap or come off).

Space maintainers

What to check

Although there is no active movement involved with a space maintainer (Figure 5.8), the usual reason for prescribing one is to prevent drifting of teeth into extraction sites while an unerupted tooth erupts into the extraction space.

Patients with space maintainers do not need to be reviewed as regularly as patients with active appliances, providing they have reliably good oral hygiene. However, patients should be reviewed at least every 3 months to confirm that:

- Oral hygiene is as good as necessary
- The appliance is still fitting adequately
- The teeth are erupting appropriately
- Sufficient space is being maintained. (Measure this at each visit and compare it with either the width of the opposite tooth should it already have erupted or with the average width of the relevant tooth. Tooth widths are shown in most standard orthodontic texts.)
- The patient is still wearing the appliance!

Trouble-shooting

Trouble-shooting with space maintainers is much more about the prevention of problems rather than the cure. Teeth can often take 6–9 months to erupt, sometimes even longer, depending on how deeply impacted they are, and it is vitally important that the patient and parent understand the importance of continuing to wear the appliance until the tooth erupts as part of the informed consent. Once space has been lost following the extraction of a permanent tooth, then it is extremely difficult to re-create it.

Next stage

Once the tooth starts to erupt, it is important that its eruption is not impeded by any acrylic, so you will need to check that this is not the case, and remove any acrylic as necessary.

If there is still no evidence that the unerupted tooth is moving in the right direction within 6 months of the space for it being created, then you may need to consider taking a radiograph of the area (periapical or sectional OPT) to check on its progress. However, radiographs may not be necessary if clinical signs suggest progress is satisfactory and these must be checked first, e.g. being able to palpate the tooth and noting that the 'bump' is heading occlusally.

Managing the end of treatment and retention

Once the teeth have moved into the desired position, it is necessary to plan phasing out the wearing of the appliance together with any retention regime.

Posterior capping

When posterior capping has been used, there will always be lateral open bites if the patient has worn the appliance as instructed. It is important that the lateral open bites are closed before the appliance wear is stopped completely as contacts between the upper and lower posterior teeth are required to stabilise the occlusion. This should be managed in the following manner:

- When the teeth are in the desired position, the posterior capping should be removed completely, but the appliance should continue to be worn on a full-time basis. Trimming the posterior capping means trimming it right down so that the occlusal surfaces are fully exposed plus approximately 2–3 mm of palatal surface, i.e. back to a normally colleted appearance. This will hold the teeth in position, but will allow the lower posterior teeth to erupt and so close the lateral open bites. Contact between upper and lower teeth is usually achieved in 6–8 weeks in a growing individual (Figure 5.9).
- Once the posterior teeth are in contact, the occlusion should retain the teeth in their new positions. However, it is important to assess this before informing the patient that they no longer need to wear their appliance.

Therefore, you are advised to check the following:

- If an anterior crossbite has been corrected, assess whether the overbite is sufficient to maintain a positive overjet. Of course, this is something that should have been determined prior to embarking on treatment, but occasionally, if the tooth is proclined a long distance, the overbite becomes minimal. In this situation, the patient will need to continue wearing the appliance for 12 hours per day (i.e. nights only) and then possibly on alternate nights until the incisors have erupted enough to establish a sufficient overbite. If little or no improvement has taken place over 2–3 months however, even if wear has been reduced to alternate nights, then the wearing of the appliance should be stopped,

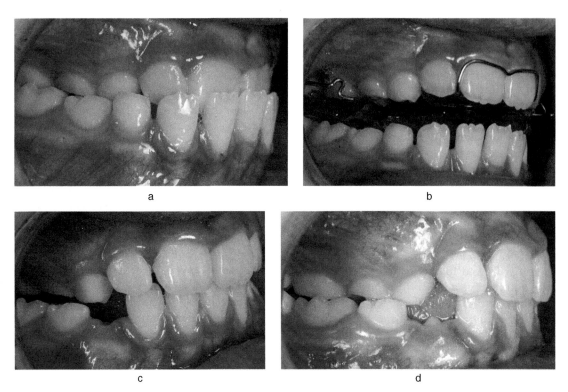

Figure 5.9 The effect of posterior capping and the effects on the posterior occlusion once it is removed. The pre-treatment occlusion (a). Posterior capping discludes the teeth so that forward movement of the upper incisors is allowed more easily (b). Once the teeth have moved over the bite, lateral open bites are apparent when the appliance is not in place (c). Therefore, the lower buccal teeth should be encouraged to erupt into occlusion by trimming off the posterior capping whilst the appliance is still worn part-time. The final occlusion without any appliance is shown (d).

accepting the likelihood of relapse. More will be said about this situation below.

- If a posterior crossbite has been corrected, assess the posterior teeth to see they are well inter-digitated in the transverse dimension in order to prevent the upper teeth tipping palatally again.
- Where teeth have been distalised, see that the posterior teeth are well inter-digitated in the antero-posterior dimension in order to prevent the upper teeth tipping mesially again.

In the last two situations above, if inter-digitation is not good, then the appliance will

need to be worn, at least part-time, until the teeth have erupted into a better occlusion.

Recreating space for the eruption of an incisor

If incisors have been distalised to allow an unerupted tooth to erupt, then the appliance will need to be worn as a passive appliance until the tooth erupts, i.e. it becomes a space maintainer. In this situation, the palatal finger springs do not need to be reactivated once the space created is large enough to allow the tooth to erupt. Once the tooth has erupted sufficiently to maintain the space for itself, then

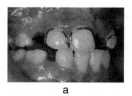 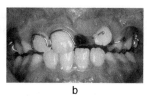 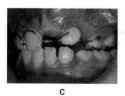 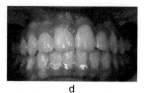

a   b   c   d

Figure 5.10 A URA being used to open space for an UL1; URC and ULC were extracted to allow space for UL2 to be retracted and to maintain the centre-line (a–c). The appliance will need to be worn as a space maintainer once sufficient space has been created and until the tooth erupts. The end result is shown (d).

wear of the appliance can be stopped (Figure 5.10).

What not to treat with standard removable appliances

Removable appliances may be used very effectively as an interceptive measure to correct the types of malocclusion indicated in the previous chapters. However, as also mentioned, accurate assessment and diagnosis of each individual case is essential because to the unwary, certain cases may appear treatable with a removable appliance, but really are not treatable with URAs. Such patients should be left alone and referred instead to a specialist orthodontist for treatment or management. The types of malocclusions that should be referred are detailed in the next section, together with the rationale for not attempting treatment with removable appliances.

Anterior crossbite with minimal overbite

If appropriately assessed, it should generally be straightforward to correct an anterior crossbite with a URA, especially if there is a mandibular displacement from an edge-to-edge incisor relationship. This correction will only be stable if the overbite (at the end of treatment) is adequate, i.e. sufficient to maintain the position of the upper incisors in front of the lower incisors.

Although before the teeth have been moved it is not possible to predict precisely the degree of overbite that will be present at the end of treatment, the degree of overbite before treatment provides a good guide. However, it is important to remember that the overbite will decrease during treatment because proclination of the upper incisors always leads to a reduction in overbite. Therefore, if the overbite is only minimal at the start, it is likely that a small anterior open bite will have been induced by the end of treatment. If there is no or only very minimal vertical overlap of the incisors or an anterior open bite at the end of treatment, the upper incisors will relapse, i.e. return to their original position as soon as the patient stops wearing the appliance (Figure 5.11).

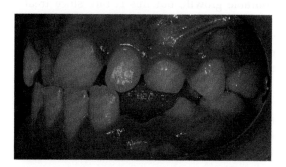

Figure 5.11 This patient has minimal overbite on UL1 so is not an ideal case to attempt correction of the anterior crossbite. If correction is attempted, the patient and parent/guardian should be fully informed of the likelihood of relapse. In addition, the oral hygiene is poor. Therefore, treatment would be contra-indicated.

It is apparent that if there is essentially complete relapse of the tooth movement achieved by the removable appliance, then the patient will have received no benefit from wearing it. However, the inherent risks of orthodontic treatment, e.g. demineralisation and root resorption, will have been present when the appliance was being worn and this will far outweigh any benefits. Therefore, treatment of cases such as this with a removable appliance should not be attempted.

Where the overbite fails to re-establish once the upper incisors have been proclined, and despite a period of part-time wear, it will have to be accepted that the appliance will have to be discontinued. It is simply not appropriate for a young patient to be expected to wear an appliance indefinitely to try to hold the upper incisors artificially. In addition to the dental health concerns that this raises, the other matter is that even if attempted, and however well intentioned, it is unlikely to be successful since no retainer or retainer wear is perfect.

In these circumstances, this should be explained to the parents/guardian. The most likely causes of such treatment failure (where a patient has been compliant and the operator has made appropriate adjustments) are incorrect diagnosis or overambitious treatment aims. Other possibilities may include unfavourable growth, but this is rare since treatment should only take approximately 3–6 months with a URA. Therefore, over such a period, the effects of growth would be expected to be relatively small.

Anterior crossbite with proclined upper incisors and/or retroclined lower incisors

In simple terms, the teeth lie in the 'neutral zone' between the muscular forces of the lips/cheeks and the tongue. This soft-tissue envelope often has a powerful effect on the position and inclination of the teeth, since the overall effect (if successful) is to get all the teeth to lie in the neutral zone, despite the skeletal discrepancy. This positioning of the teeth by the soft tissues in malocclusions resulting from a skeletal discrepancy is often referred to as soft-tissue compensation.

In Class III cases, soft-tissue compensation results in proclination of the upper incisors, retroclination of the lower incisors, or both. Therefore, the tooth position may mask significant skeletal discrepancies (Figure 5.12).

It is essential that the amount of soft-tissue compensation for the skeletal pattern is fully considered when treatment planning a case with an anterior crossbite. To the unwary or inexperienced, at first glance, these malocclusions may appear to be correctable with a URA, as described in Chapter 3. It is often possible to assess the inclination of the incisor teeth clinically, but, in cases where there is a more significant skeletal component to the malocclusion, the most appropriate way is to analyse a lateral cephalogram. Therefore, the input from a specialist orthodontist is required.

If the upper incisors are already proclined and/or the lower incisors are retroclined, there is very little scope for further compensation by the incisors for the skeletal discrepancy. This is because when the teeth are not positioned at the correct inclination, the occlusal forces are not transmitted down the long axis of the teeth. This is referred to as non-axial loading and can lead to movement of the teeth in a labio-lingual direction each time the upper and lower teeth occlude. This, in turn, causes flexing of the alveolar bone. These so-called 'jiggling' forces can potentially damage both the root of the tooth (causing root resorption) and the periodontium, especially in the presence of plaque. In addition, the appearance is likely to be very unaesthetic.

Severe skeletal Class III

For patients with a severe Class III skeletal discrepancy, the only way to potentially achieve a positive overjet with a URA is to excessively

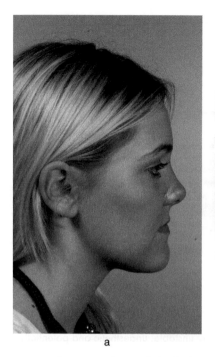

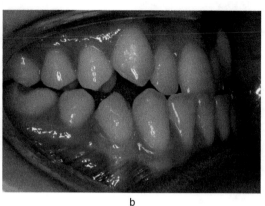

b

a

Figure 5.12 This patient has a skeletal Class III pattern (a) but soft-tissue compensation camouflages (masks) this to an extent: the teeth are compensating for the Class III base, resulting in proclination of the upper incisors, and retroclination of the lower incisors (b).

procline the upper incisor teeth. As discussed in the previous section, this can have deleterious effects on the supporting structures of the teeth and should be avoided. It will also look unacceptable.

Furthermore, a severe Class III skeletal discrepancy present in the mixed dentition, prior to the patient starting the adolescent growth spurt, is likely to become significantly worse during the growth spurt. This is because the mandible grows more and for longer than the maxilla during adolescence (Figure 5.13).

Class II division 1 malocclusion with upright upper incisors

Soft-tissue compensation in Class II cases leads to uprighting/retroclination of the upper incisors and proclination of the lower incisors. Nevertheless, there may still be an increased

overjet even with the soft-tissue compensation (Figure 5.14).

Although it is possible to camouflage these cases, i.e. create a Class I occlusion on a Class II skeletal base, an aesthetic result requires torqueing movements of the teeth and this can only be achieved with a fixed appliance. Treating cases such as this with a removable appliance leads to retroclination of the upper incisors with a consequent increase in overbite and in the amount of gingival show. This combination of features may lead to a very unaesthetic outcome and potential gingival trauma, depending on the depth of the overbite.

Severe skeletal class II

In the past, even malocclusions with a severe Class II skeletal pattern were treated by extraction of the upper first premolars followed by

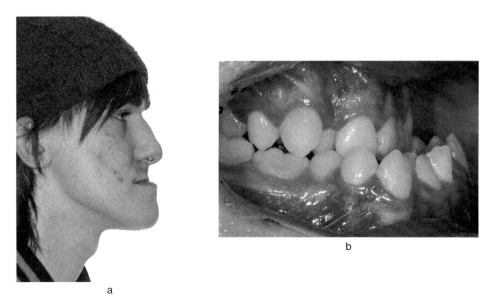

Figure 5.13 This patient has a severe Class III skeletal pattern with marked dento-alveolar compensation, particularly in the lower arch. Any attempt to correct the Class III incisor relationship with a URA would lead to excessive proclination of the upper incisors, which would be highly unstable, unaesthetic and potentially damaging to the teeth.

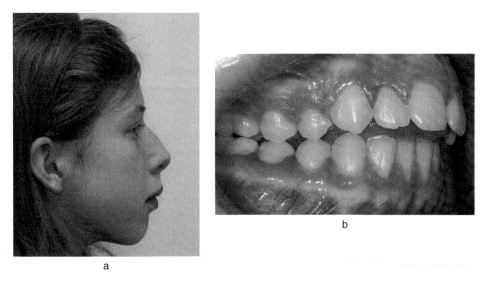

Figure 5.14 A patient with a moderate skeletal Class II pattern and upright upper incisors where URA treatment would be contra-indicated as the upper incisors would be retroclined, leading to a very unaesthetic appearance (a and b). The result would also be very unstable as the upper incisors could procline again, leading to a re-opening of any extraction spaces. (The overbite is reduced in this case, so it is unlikely to deepen to the extent of becoming traumatic.)

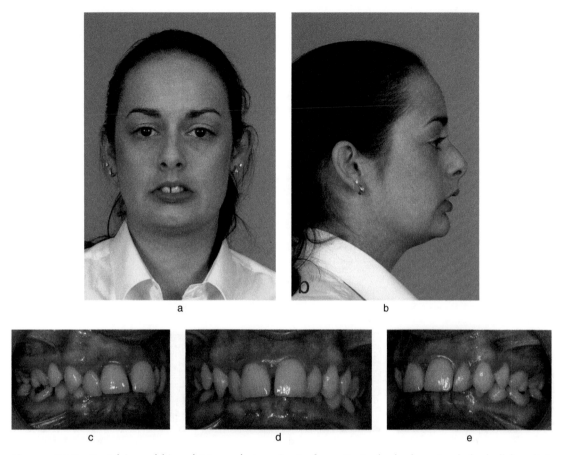

Figure 5.15 Facial (a and b) and intra-oral views (c–e) of a patient who had previously had all four first premolars extracted and two courses of URA treatment to correct the severe Class II division 1. As can be seen, this treatment has relapsed on both occasions, leaving the patient with a spaced ULS, the appearance of which concerned her. An attempt has been made to disguise this with veneers on the upper incisors which, in combination with fair oral health, are causing gingivitis. The deep overbite has been exacerbated by the extraction of the lower first premolars and the subsequent retroclination of the lower incisors.

retroclination of the upper incisors with a removable appliance (Figure 5.15).

There are two main problems with this type of treatment:

- The end result is unaesthetic due to the overjet still being increased (despite the retroclination of the upper incisors), spacing and the frequent increase in gingival show.
- Because of the limitations of tooth movement with a removable appliance, in cases

with a severe Class II skeletal pattern, it is often not possible to fully reduce the overjet with tipping movements alone. In these circumstances, the upper incisors do not fall under lower lip control at the end of treatment and, because of this, the upper incisors procline again once retention is stopped. As the upper incisors procline, the lower lip is able to function behind them again, proclining them further and re-opening the spaces that were created when the upper first

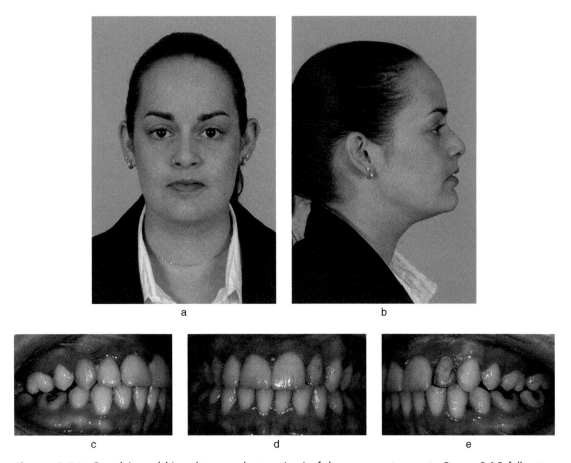

a   b

c   d   e

Figure 5.16 Facial (a and b) and intra-oral views (c–e) of the same patient as in Figure 5.15 following treatment with upper and lower fixed appliances and bimaxillary orthognathic surgery. These photographs were taken at the time of removal of the fixed appliances. Oral health requires some improvement and the veneer on UL2 needs to be replaced. The upper incisors are now under lower lip control and the reduction of the overjet will be stable.

premolars were extracted. The end result is even less aesthetic than the appearance at the start of treatment, because not only has the overjet returned, but the upper labial segment will now be spaced. Many cases treated in this way in the past are now seen by specialist orthodontists and require repeat treatment, this time with fixed appliances and further extractions and/or orthognathic surgery. Such treatment takes 2–3 years, but in some cases the patient's treatment may be totally compromised or even

rendered impossible if, for example, significant root resorption and/or other dental disease occurred during the previous treatment (Figures 5.15 and 5.16).

Patients with a severe Class II skeletal pattern should always be referred to a specialist orthodontist before the adolescent growth spurt (preferably at age 9–10 years for girls and 11–12 years for boys) before any treatment is attempted.

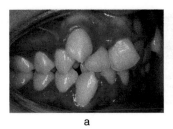 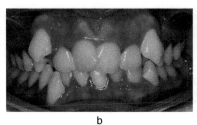 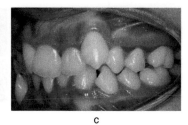

a   b   c

Figure 5.17   Intra-oral views of a Class I malocclusion showing severe crowding with buccally displaced and disto-angular upper canine teeth (a–c). URA treatment following extraction of the upper first premolars is inappropriate in this case due to the angulation of the canine teeth, which would worsen during URA treatment.

Buccal canines that are distally tipped pre-treatment Figure 5.17)

As stated in Chapter 2, the only type of tooth movement that a removable appliance can perform is tipping of the teeth. As teeth are moved distally, they will be tipped distally. Whilst this is acceptable if the tooth was mesially tipped pre-treatment, further distal tipping of a canine that is already distally tipped leads to a very unaesthetic result.

Also, the angulation of a tooth provides a strong clue as to the root position. In a buccal canine that is mesially tipped, the root apex will be distal to the position of the crown. Therefore, tipping the crown of the tooth distally will act to improve the tooth's ability to withstand occlusal forces and is likely to be stable as the root of the canine tooth will become more parallel to the roots of the surrounding teeth.

In a canine that is distally angulated, the apex of the root will be in a more mesial position. Therefore, not only will further distal tipping of this tooth be unsightly, also it will be less stable and potentially deleterious in terms of the tooth being able to withstand occlusal load.

Canines that need to be retracted, but are already distally angulated, require significant movement of the root through the bone and this type of tooth movement can only be performed by fixed appliances.

Crowded cases

Cases that are moderately/severely crowded often require extraction of permanent teeth to create space for alignment of the remaining teeth.

When teeth have been extracted, it is essential that the space is closed by bodily movement of the teeth on either side of the extraction space. This is because in order to keep the extraction space closed, the roots of the teeth that have been moved need to be parallel to each other at the end of treatment.

Removable appliances are only able to tip teeth into extraction spaces and, therefore, at the end of treatment, even if the space has been closed, tipped teeth will upright again, re-opening the extraction sites to a greater or lesser degree.

Bodily movement of teeth requires the use of fixed appliances, hence referral to an orthodontist trained in the use of fixed appliances is necessary (Figure 5.18).

Tooth malalignment that cannot be corrected with tipping movements

It is fair to say that the definitive correction of the great majority of malocclusions cannot be achieved with removable appliances. This is because definitive correction that provides a functional, aesthetic and stable result will,

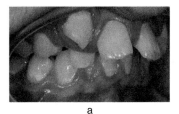
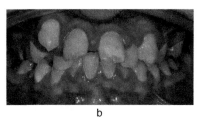
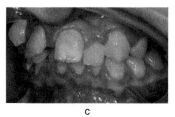

a   b   c

Figure 5.18 Intra-oral views of a patient with a Class II division 1 malocclusion and severe crowding in UR2, UR3 region and an upper centre-line shift to the right (a–c). UR3 is disto-angular. Bodily movement of teeth is required to align them, and correct root position and the upper centre-line. Therefore, fixed appliances are required for the full correction of this malocclusion.

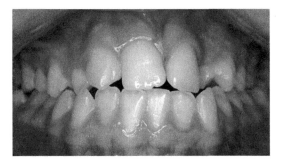

Figure 5.19 Malocclusion with missing UR2 and UL2, palatally ectopic UL3 and large upper centre-line shift to the left. There is also an edge-to-edge relationship of the incisors. Bodily movement is required to correct the centre-line shift and torqueing movements will be required to bring UL3 into alignment from its current palatal position. Only a fixed appliance should be used to treat this malocclusion.

almost always, require tooth movements other than tipping movements alone (Figure 5.19).

De-rotating teeth, bodily movement and torqueing movements of roots and/or crowns of teeth all require a force couple and three-dimensional control that can only be achieved with the use of a full-sized rectangular wire in a bracket slot.

When to refer

All dental healthcare professionals responsible for the treatment of patients, no matter what their role, need to have a detailed knowledge of the eruption dates and eruption sequence of both the primary (deciduous) and secondary (permanent) teeth, and of the important stages in occlusal development. If you do not know these facts, then you will not be able to detect when there is a problem with tooth eruption/ occlusal development. The significance of this is that a delay in diagnosis may result in your patient requiring significantly more involved treatment than would have been necessary if the problem had been detected at the optimal time. An increasing number of general dental practitioners are now being sued by parents of patients for misdiagnosis/failure of diagnosis of eruption and problems in occlusal development. Do ensure that you are aware of the necessary information that is covered in detail in a number of undergraduate orthodontic texts.

The optimal times and some common reasons for referral in a patient exhibiting the average age for tooth eruption are:

- If a permanent tooth has not started to erupt within 6 months of its antimere starting to erupt, or the sequence of eruption is altered/ asymmetric, then radiographic investigation is necessary to exclude a pathological reason for the non-eruption. If pathology/supernumerary teeth/ectopic development position are detected radiographically, then a referral to a specialist orthodontist is necessary.

- All children should have their upper permanent canine teeth palpated in the upper buccal sulcus by the age of 10 years. If these teeth are not palpable and the primary teeth are firm, then it is necessary to undertake radiographic examination using the parallax technique to detect whether the upper permanent canines are ectopic. These teeth are ectopic in about 2% of the population, i.e. 1 in 50 of your patients.
- Many patients with a severe Class II division 1 malocclusion would benefit from the use of a functional appliance (see Chapter 10). These need to be used during the adolescent growth spurt. Obviously, there is variability in the age at which children experience this, but on average girls experience this approximately 2 years ahead of boys. Girls with Class II division 1 malocclusions need to be referred by the age of 10 years to ensure that the growth spurt is not missed, but boys may be referred at the age of 12–13 years. However, all children with severe Class II division 1 malocclusions should be encouraged to wear a mouth guard when playing sport as their upper incisor teeth are at an increased risk of trauma.
- Rarely, if a Class III malocclusion is due to a hypoplastic maxilla (see Chapter 10), patients may be treated around the age of 8 years, and so require an early referral. Successful treatment cannot however be guaranteed. Furthermore, many Class III cases more frequently have a prognathic mandible and will not be definitively treated until mandibular growth has ceased, around 15–16 years of age in girls and 17–18 years in boys. This is because a significant worsening of a Class III malocclusion can take place during the adolescent growth spurt and the definitive treatment may differ significantly, depending on the amount of mandibular growth that occurs.

The above is of course not a comprehensive list of patients who may benefit from early referral, but does highlight some examples where removable appliance treatment of some form or another may be helpful.

Referral to a specialist orthodontist

Once you have decided that you require advice regarding the diagnosis of a malocclusion or you consider that the malocclusion requires specialist treatment, e.g. using fixed appliances, then you should refer the patient to a suitably qualified clinician who will be able to provide advice and treatment as required. In the UK, but also elsewhere, referral is affected by the criteria of the Index of Orthodontic Treatment Need (IOTN). This should therefore also be borne in mind.

It is your responsibility, as the referring practitioner, to ensure that the healthcare professional you are referring to has the appropriate knowledge and skills to be able to provide your patient with an acceptable level of care. You can be sued for breach of contract in your duty of care to your patient if it can be demonstrated that you referred to an individual who does not have the knowledge or the skill to treat a malocclusion and the patient suffers harm because of this.

As stated in Chapter 2, it is essential that all patients are dentally fit; have received dietary advice to which they are adhering; and have excellent oral health before referral to an orthodontist. All appliances, especially fixed appliances, pose a significant risk to dental health if used in the wrong oral environment (Figure 5.20).

Information to include in the referral letter

A 'please see and treat' letter is never appropriate and may well be returned to you with a request for more information before the referral is accepted. The orthodontist will require enough information to be able to make an informed judgement regarding:

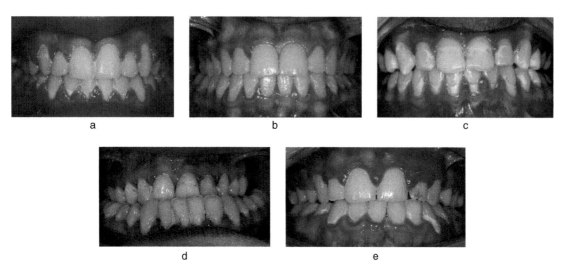

Figure 5.20 Examples of individuals who did not maintain excellent oral health and dietary control during treatment with fixed appliances (a–e). Demineralisation lesions are most often seen on the cervical aspect of the upper incisors and lower canines and first premolars. The poor gingival health is evident. It is also evident that some of these cases have had the appliances removed early, prior to completion of orthodontic treatment, in order to protect the teeth and gingivae from any further damage caused by wearing fixed appliances.

- The urgency of the referral
- The suitability of the patient for orthodontic treatment
- Whether the malocclusion is suitable for treatment by that particular orthodontist/ practice (based on IOTN).

Therefore, all letters of referral should contain the following information:

- Patient's name, address, postcode, age and date of birth, and full, accurate, contact details
- Reason for the referral and what the patient's complaint is
- Patient's medical history
- How long they have been a patient with you and whether they attend regularly for routine check-ups
- The standard of the oral hygiene; whether oral hygiene instruction and dietary advice has been given and adhered to
- Previous dental treatment including restorations and extractions, and how tolerant the patient was of treatment; report any previous orthodontic treatment

- Any history of trauma to the facial region or the teeth
- Any pertinent social history
- Motivation for treatment, whether any other family members have received orthodontic treatment and where this treatment was provided
- Precise summary of the malocclusion including:
  - Skeletal and relevant soft-tissue pattern
  - Stage of occlusal development
  - Teeth present/absent
  - Crowding/spacing
  - Incisor and molar relationship
  - Measurement of overjet and assessment of overbite
  - Presence of a mandibular displacement
  - Radiographic features including pathology
  - Highlight any teeth of poor prognosis
  - The IOTN.

A copy/print out of any recent/relevant radiographs should always be included with the letter, as should any study models that have been taken.

Example of referral letter

Dear Mr Wire,

Re: Ann Other, DOB 12/03/02
      Telephone: 01011 222333
      1A Street, Any Town
      Countyshire, AT1 2ZX

I would be very grateful if you could arrange to see Ann regarding her severe Class II division 1 malocclusion. Ann is being teased at school and is reluctant to smile because her top teeth 'stick out'.

Ann and her family are new patients to me, but have been regular attenders at this practice for many years. Her oral hygiene is generally of a very good standard, but I have recently given some oral health instruction in relation to the first molars. She has not had any experience of dental treatment in the past and is currently dentally fit. Medically, she has mild asthma, for which she takes a salbutamol inhaler when required. Ann and her mum are very keen for her to have treatment and understand what is involved with orthodontic treatment as Ann's older brother had treatment at your practice a couple of years ago.

In summary, Ann is 10 years old and has a Class II division 1 malocclusion on a moderate Class II skeletal base with decreased vertical proportions and incompetent lips with a lower lip trap. Intra-orally she is in the normal early permanent dentition for her age. The lower arch is well aligned and the upper labial segment is proclined and spaced. In occlusion, the overjet is increased to 12 mm and the overbite is increased and complete to palate. The molar relationship is a full unit Class II bilaterally. There are no crossbites and no displacement of the mandible. I have not taken any radiographs as there has been no clinical justification.

I understand from Mrs Other that Ann has been growing rapidly for the last 12 months and so I would be very grateful if you could see her with some urgency in case she requires a functional appliance to correct her malocclusion.

Many thanks in anticipation of your help with Ann's orthodontic treatment.

Yours sincerely

Test Yourself

In this chapter, clinical cases will be shown and readers will be asked to decide whether use of an upper removable appliance (URA) is sensible or not and, if it is, to design an appropriate appliance. At the end of the chapter, the answers will be given and line drawings provided of a possible appliance design where appropriate. In some cases, more than one design may be feasible. If URA treatment is not appropriate, the reasons will be explained.

Learning outcomes

At the end of this chapter you should have increased your knowledge and understanding of:

- When the use of a URA may be appropriate
- When the use of a URA may be inappropriate
- How appliances should be drawn and written on a laboratory card

---

Note that in these cases, it is assumed that any suggested treatment could *only* be undertaken once a full clinical examination had taken place and all necessary records had been examined by the operator. This would, of course, also include the necessary and appropriate radiographic and study model examination. The following cases are therefore intended only to give examples of what might be possible and where treatment should be avoided and/or a specialist opinion sought.

Note also that in all the mixed dentition cases that follow, and where the upper permanent canines are unerupted, that they are palpable buccally.

Orthodontic Retainers and Removable Appliances: Principles of Design and Use, First Edition.
Friedy Luther and Zararna Nelson-Moon.
© 2013 Friedy Luther and Zararna Nelson-Moon. Published 2013 by Blackwell Publishing Ltd.

Questions

Case 1 (Figure 6.1)

This patient is 11 years old and has no complaints, but her mother is concerned about the crossbite of UR1. She has also noticed that LR1 is being displaced labially. There is a forward displacement on closure associated with the incisor crossbite and the patient is fit and well.

Carry out an orthodontic assessment of the patient and then answer the following question:

1. Do you think this patient's UR1, which is in crossbite, is suitable for correction using a URA?

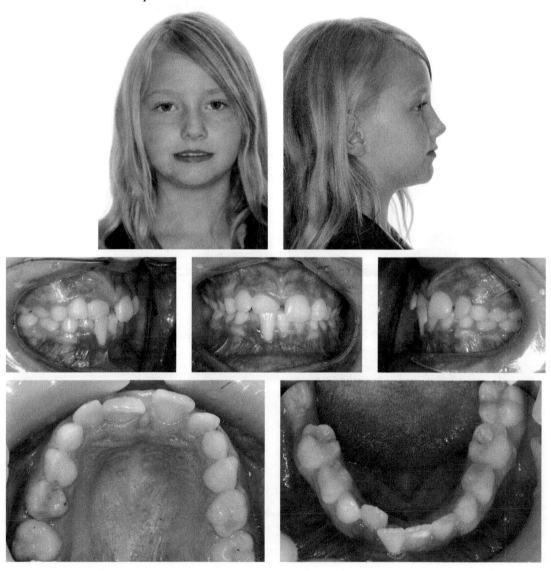

Figure 6.1   Facial and intra-oral views of Case 1.

Case 2 (Figure 6.2)

This male patient is 11 years old and is concerned that his front teeth stick out. He has not had orthodontic treatment before. He is fit and well.

Carry out an orthodontic assessment of this patient and then answer the following questions:

1. Is the patient suitable for correction of his malocclusion using a URA with the extraction of the upper first premolar teeth? If so, design a suitable appliance.
2. What would you need to achieve at the end of treatment to ensure stability?

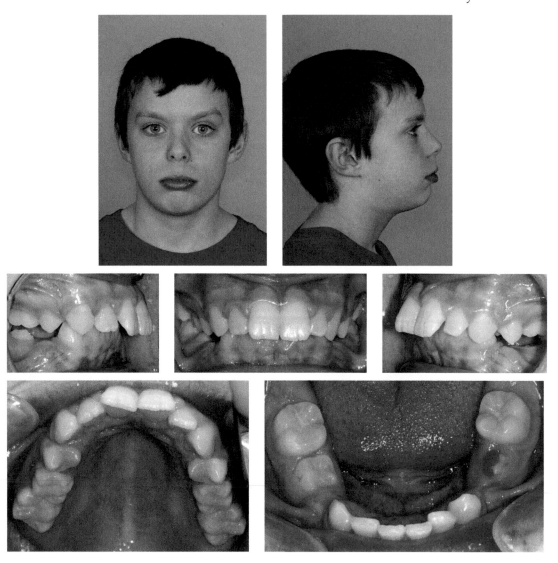

Figure 6.2 Facial and intra-oral views of Case 2.

Case 3 (Figure 6.3)

This 12-year-old boy is concerned regarding his bite. He has a mandibular displacement anteriorly from an edge-to-edge incisor relationship. He is fit and well.

Carry out an orthodontic assessment of this patient and then answer the following questions:

1. Would you use a URA to correct the anterior crossbite? If so, design the appliance.
2. Would you use a URA to correct the crossbite of UL6? If so, design the appliance.

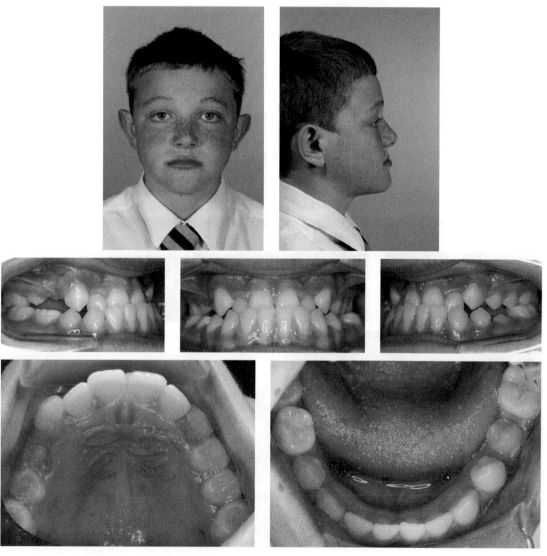

Figure 6.3   Facial and intra-oral views of Case 3.

Case 4 (Figure 6.4)

This patient complains of crooked teeth. She is 13 years old and is fit and well.

Carry out an orthodontic assessment of this patient and then answer the following question:

1. Do you think this patient's UR3, which is in crossbite, is suitable for correction using a URA?

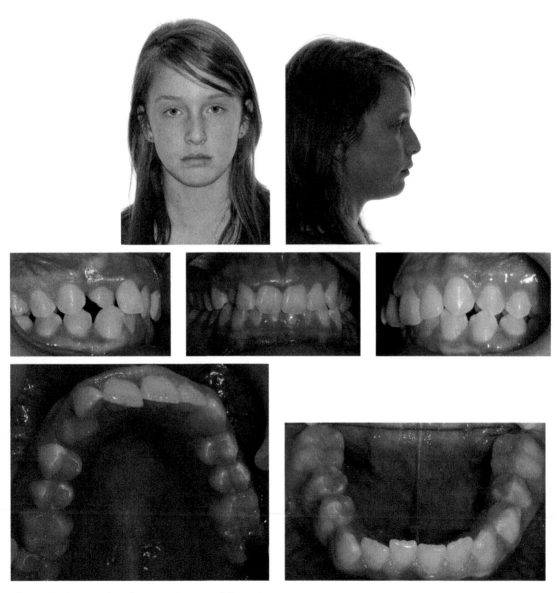

Figure 6.4 Facial and intra-oral views of Case 4.

Case 5 (Figure 6.5)

This patient is 9 years old and has no complaints, but her mother is concerned about the crossbite of UR2. There is a displacement on closure associated with the incisor crossbite. The patient is fit and well.

Carry out an orthodontic assessment of this patient and then answer the following question:

1. Do you think this patient's UR2, which is in crossbite, is suitable for correction using a URA?

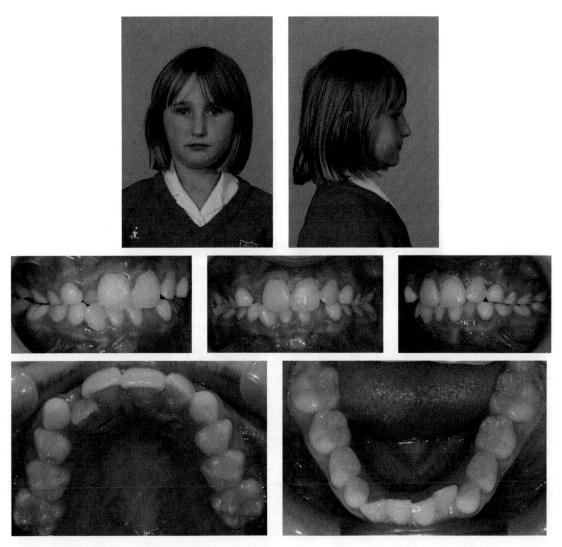

Figure 6.5 Facial and intra-oral views of Case 5.

Case 6 (Figure 6.6)

This 24-year-old female patient is concerned about the appearance of her front teeth. She has had some orthodontic intervention before, which involved the extraction of UR4, LL4 and LR4, but no appliance treatment. She is fit and well.

Carry out an orthodontic assessment of this patient and then answer the following questions:

1. Could a URA be used to decrease the overjet after extraction of UL4? If so, design the appliance.
2. Could a URA be used to correct the upper centre-line after extraction of UL4? If so, design the appliance.
3. What other aspect of the malocclusion could a URA be used to treat? Design the appliance.

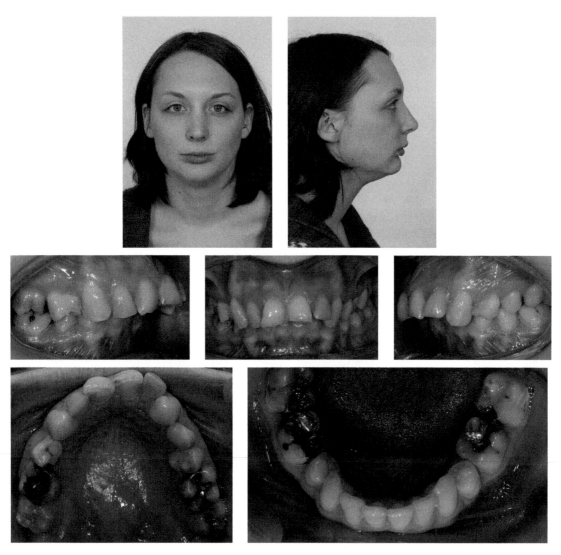

Figure 6.6   Facial and intra-oral views of Case 6.

Case 7 (Figure 6.7)

This 8-year-old patient was referred by his dentist regarding the posterior crossbite. The patient himself has no concerns and is fit and well. He has a mandibular displacement to the left of more than 2 mm off ULC.

Carry out an orthodontic assessment of this patient and then answer the following question:

1. Would you use a URA to correct the posterior crossbite and/or UL2 position? If so, design a URA(s).

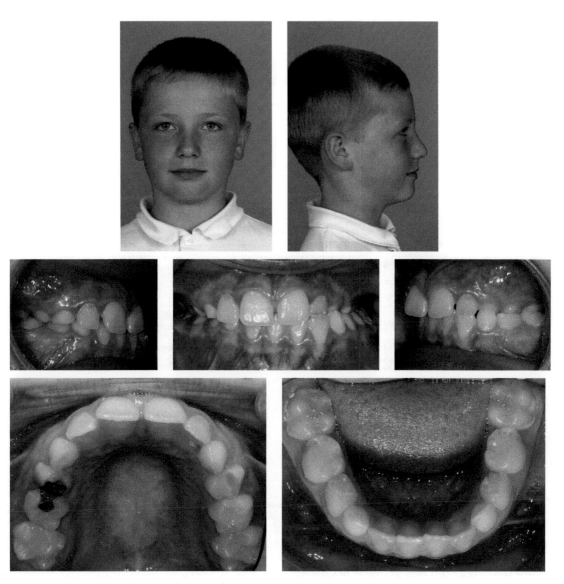

Figure 6.7 Facial and intra-oral views of Case 7.

Case 8 (Figure 6.8)

This patient is 8 years old and has no complaint, but his parents are concerned by his crooked teeth biting the wrong way round. There is a displacement on closure associated with the incisor crossbite. The patient is fit and well.

Carry out an orthodontic assessment of this patient and then answer the following question:

1. Do you think the patient is suitable for URA treatment to push the upper right central and lateral incisor over the bite?

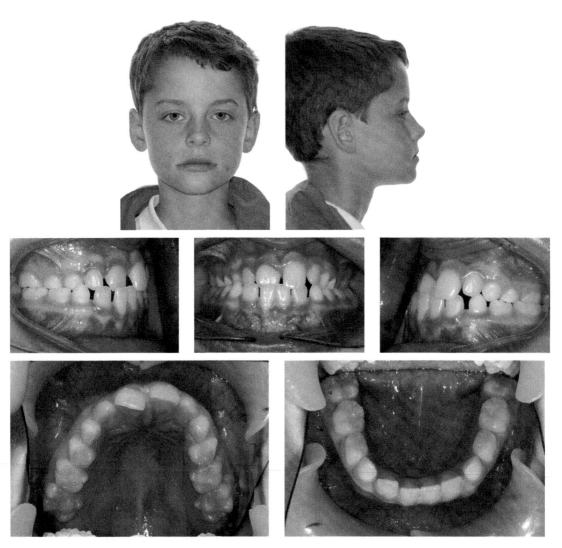

Figure 6.8 Facial and intra-oral views of Case 8.

Case 9 (Figure 6.9)

This 9-year-old patient has previously had a supernumerary tooth removed which was preventing the eruption of UR1. UR1 has not erupted any further for the past 6 months. The patient is concerned regarding the appearance of UR1. She is fit and well.

Carry out an orthodontic assessment of this patient and then answer the following question:

1. Could a URA be used to bring UR1 down into a more ideal position? If so, design the URA.

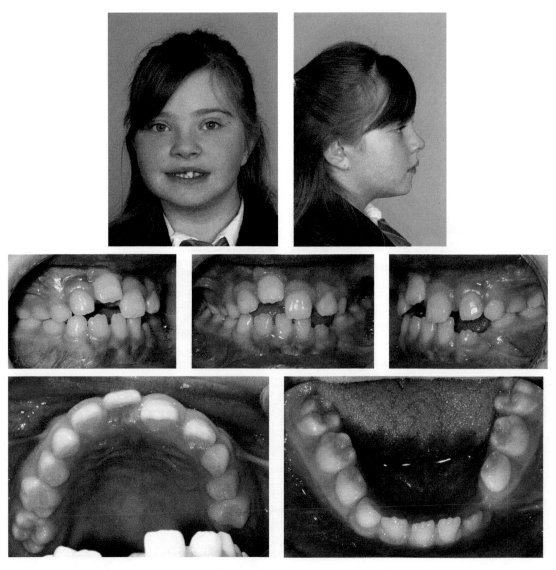

Figure 6.9   Facial and intra-oral views of Case 9.

Case 10 (Figure 6.10)

This patient is 8 years old and does not like the appearance of her top front teeth. The patient is fit and well.

Carry out an orthodontic assessment of this patient and then answer the following question:

1. What is the cause of this patient's malocclusion? Do you think this patient's malocclusion is suitable for treatment using a URA?

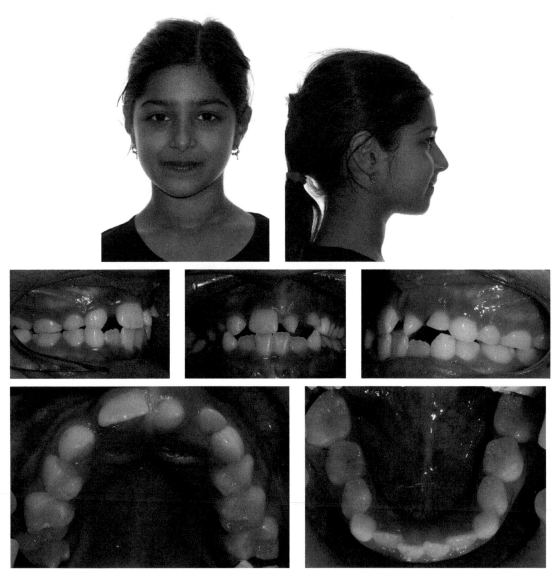

Figure 6.10 Facial and intra-oral views of Case 10.

Case 11 (Figure 6.11)

This patient complains of crooked teeth. She is 13 years old and is fit and well. There is no displacement on closure.

Carry out an orthodontic assessment of this patient and then answer the following questions:

1. Do you think the patient is suitable for URA space maintenance to allow spontaneous alignment of both the upper canines following loss of both upper first premolars? If she is suitable, design the appliance.
2. Could a URA be used to align the buccally crowded canines following loss of UR4 and UL4? If she is suitable, design the appliance.
3. Do you think the patient is suitable for a URA to correct the upper lateral incisor crossbite? If she is suitable, design the appliance.

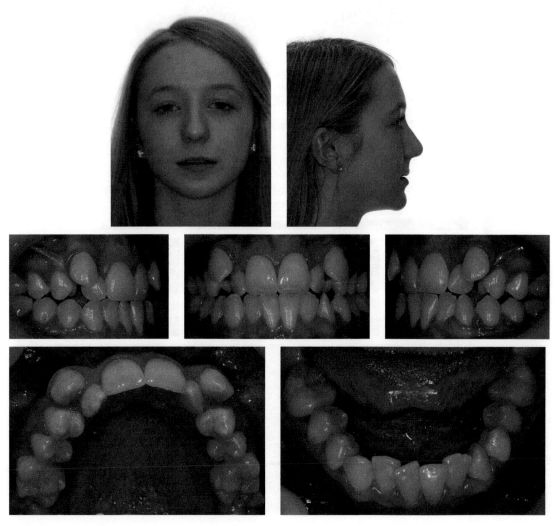

Figure 6.11 Facial and intra-oral views of Case 11.

Case 12 (Figure 6.12)

This 8-year-old girl was referred by her dentist because UR1 has not erupted, although it is palpable high in the labial sulcus. She is fit and well.

Carry out an orthodontic assessment of this patient and then answer the following questions:

1. Would you use a URA to re-create the space for UR1 to erupt? If so, design the appliance.
2. Would you advocate the removal of any teeth prior to activating any appliance you might use?

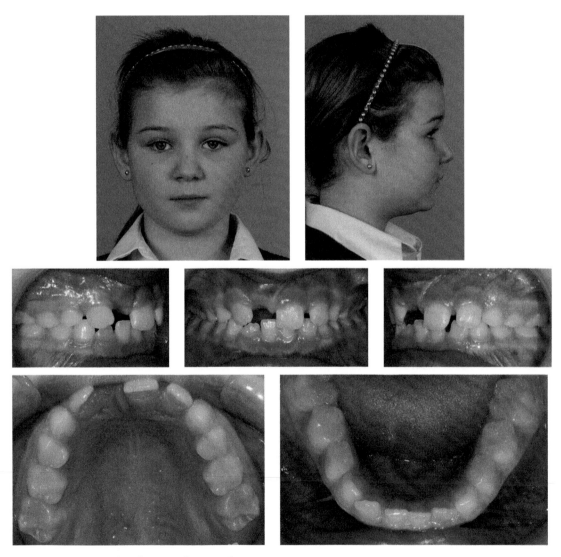

Figure 6.12   Facial and intra-oral views of Case 12.

Case 13 (Figure 6.13)

This patient is 11 years old and is concerned about his bite. He has had some orthodontic treatment with a URA before. He does not have a mandibular displacement and he is aware that oral hygiene needs to improve significantly prior to any orthodontic treatment being provided.

Carry out an orthodontic assessment of this patient and then answer the following questions:

1. Assuming that oral hygiene improves to the required standard, would you use a URA to hold open the space for the unerupted upper permanent canine teeth following extraction of the upper first premolar teeth? If so, design the appliance.
2. Could a URA be used to correct the upper centre-line shift? If so, design the appliance.
3. Could a URA be used to correct the anterior crossbite? If so, design the appliance.
4. Could a URA be used to correct the posterior crossbites? If so, design the appliance.

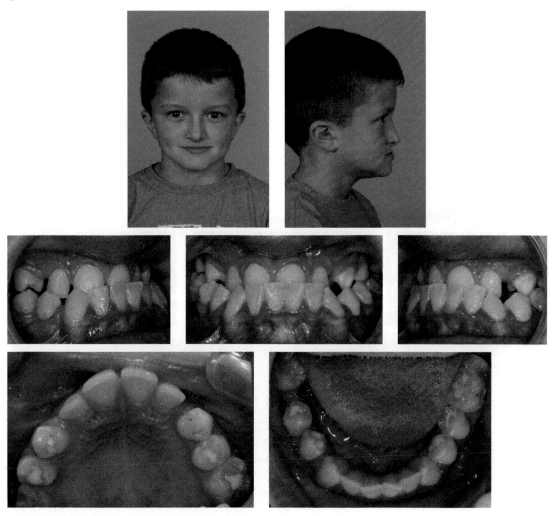

Figure 6.13 Facial and intra-oral views of Case 13.

Case 14 (Figure 6.14)

This patient is 8 years old and complains that you cannot see his top front tooth. There is a displacement on closure associated with the incisor crossbite. He is fit and well.

Carry out an orthodontic assessment of this patient and then answer the following question:

1. What is the cause of this patient's malocclusion? Do you think this patient's malocclusion is suitable for correction using a URA?

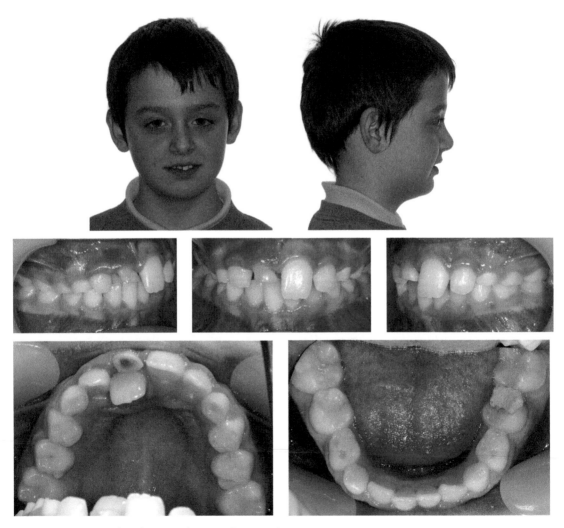

Figure 6.14 Facial and intra-oral views of Case 14.

Case 15 (Figure 6.15)

This 12-year-old female patient is concerned about the prominence of her upper front teeth. She is fit and well.

Carry out an orthodontic assessment of this patient and then answer the following question:

1. Could this patient be treated by extraction of upper first premolars and URA(s) to retract the upper canines and then reduce the overjet? If so, design the URA(s).

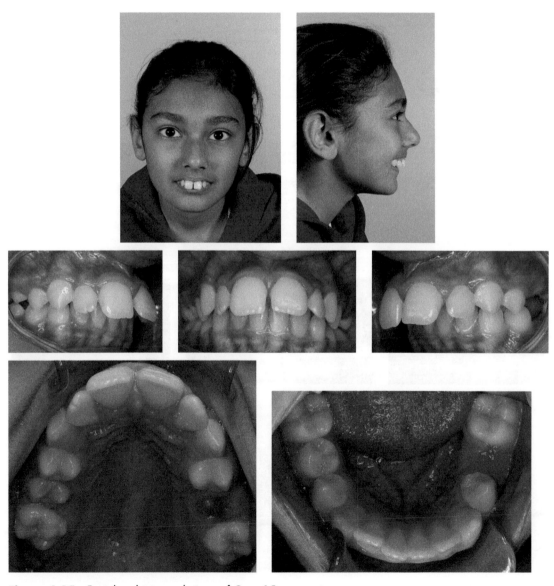

Figure 6.15 Facial and intra-oral views of Case 15.

Case 16 (Figure 6.16)

This 11-year-old girl is concerned regarding the position of her front teeth. She is fit and well and has a mandibular displacement from an edge-to-edge incisor relationship.

Carry out an orthodontic assessment of this patient and then answer the following question:

1. Would you use a URA to correct the position of the upper central incisors? If so, design an appliance.

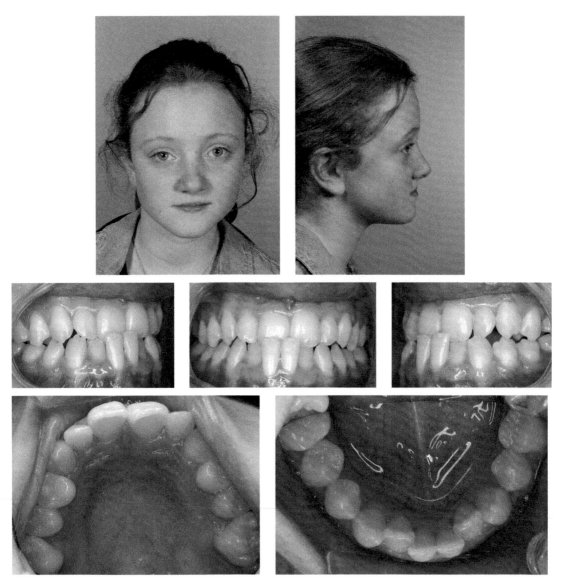

Figure 6.16   Facial and intra-oral views of Case 16.

Answers

Note that in the cases in whom URAs are advocated for interceptive treatment, it is assumed that the patient will have improved their oral hygiene to the necessary standard, that there is dietary control and that any carious lesions have been restored.

The rationale for the design of the appliances is detailed in Chapter 3 and is not repeated here. However, the reader is advised to review the relevant sections as appropriate.

Case 1

Orthodontic assessment

This patient has a Class I skeletal pattern with average vertical proportions, no facial asymmetry, but mildly incompetent lips.

The patient is in the mixed dentition and has mild gingivitis around the LLS and some recession associated with LR1. There is also evidence of caries in some deciduous teeth and LR6 has previously been extracted.

The arches are well aligned except for the irregularity associated with UR1 and LR1, and the mild rotation of UL2 (disto-labial). The ULS and LLS are normally inclined clinically except for UR1 (retroclined) and LR1 (proclined).

In occlusion, the incisor relationship is Class I except for UR1 where the relationship is Class III. The overjet is within normal limits except for UR1 (–1 mm). The overbite is average and complete to tooth; the centre-lines are co-incident and correct. The lower centre-line is marginally to the right.

The buccal segment relationship is Class I on the left, but LR6 has previously been removed. There is a slight forward displacement on closure associated with UR1 and LR1.

Problem list

- Mild gingivitis and recession in the lower labial segment (LLS)
- Caries

- Mother concerned about crossbite and displacement of LR1
- Mandibular displacement
- Rotated UL2
- Crossbite of UR1
- Labially displaced LR1

Answers to questions

1. Suitable for removable appliance treatment to push UR1 over the bite?
   Yes.

Rationale: The patient has a favourable skeletal pattern; there is a forward displacement on closure (the patient can make an edge-to-edge contact of UR1 with LR1), and the overbite will be favourable once the eruption of UR1 is no longer impeded by the occlusion and LR1 and LR2 are able to spontaneously align. The incisor inclinations are favourable and there is room to move the tooth.

It is important to note that prior to treatment starting, the patient and parent/guardian should be warned that the overjet may increase following correction of UR1 as the displacement is corrected. The mandible may therefore drop back as it no longer has to be brought forward (displaced forward) to 'clear' the instanding UR1.

Appliance design
A suggested design is shown in Figure 6.17.

Case 2

Orthodontic assessment

The patient has a severe Class II division 1 malocclusion on a moderate Class II skeletal base with an increased lower anterior face height and an increased Frankfort–mandibular planes angle (FMPA). The mandible is symmetrical. The lips are incompetent and the naso-labial angle is average.

Intra-orally, the patient is in the late mixed dentition phase with both upper second primary

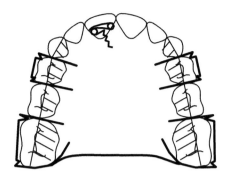

Please construct an upper removable appliance to procline UR1:

1. Z-spring UR1 – 0.5 mm hard ss wire

2. Adams' clasps UR6, UL6 – 0.7 mm hard ss wire

3. Adams' clasps URD, ULD – 0.6 mm hard ss wire

4. ½ occlusal coverage posterior capping UR6 – URC and ULC – UL6

Figure 6.17   Laboratory prescription for a URA to procline UR1 (Case 1).

molar teeth retained. The LLS is mildly crowded and of average inclination, and the ULS is also mildly crowded, but proclined.

In occlusion, the overjet is increased (10 mm) and the overbite is increased and complete to gingivae.

The buccal segment relationship is a full unit Class II on the molars and canines bilaterally. The upper centre-line is coincident with the facial midline and the lower centre-line is 1 mm to the right of the upper centre-line. There are no crossbites and no displacements.

Problem list

- Patient's complaint: top teeth stick out
- Moderate skeletal Class II base
- Incompetent lips and lower lip trap
- Mild crowding of LLS
- Proclination of upper labial segment (ULS)
- Increased overjet
- Increased and complete overbite
- Class II buccal segment relationship

Answers to questions

1. Suitable for treatment with a URA and extraction of upper first premolars?
   No.

Rationale: The patient has a moderate Class II skeletal pattern with a retrognathic mandible and, therefore, the Class II division 1 incisor relationship is not so much due to the position of the upper incisors, but more due to the mandible being set back. The marked puckering over the chin caused by activity of the mentalis muscle indicates that the lips are incompetent at rest and the proclination of the upper incisors would suggest that there is a lower lip trap. The naso-labial angle is average, further confirming that the maxilla and upper teeth are in the correct position.

As URAs are only able to tip teeth, retracting the upper canines into the space created by extraction of the upper first premolars would cause them to become very distally tipped as they are already at an ideal angulation and would need to move by the whole width of a premolar (7 mm). Distally angulated canines are unaesthetic and tipping a tooth to this extent is prone to relapse, which would lead to re-opening of the extraction space and an increase in the overjet.

Although the upper incisors are proclined pre-treatment, overjet correction will only be stable if the upper incisors are brought under lower lip control. Reducing the overjet to this extent with a URA would excessively retrocline the upper incisors and turn a Class II division 1 malocclusion into a Class II division 2 malocclusion at the end of treatment. Retroclination of the upper incisors to this extent may also cause the upper lip to drop back, accentuating the nose and causing the lower part of the face to slope backwards from nose to chin.

As the patient has incompetent lips, the upper incisor position will not be retained by the lower lip. Any relapse of the upper incisor position will allow the lower lip to get behind the upper incisors again, further proclining them until they have returned to their original position. Because two teeth have now been removed from the upper arch, relapse of the upper incisor position will cause spacing of these teeth, potentially leaving the patient with a malocclusion that is worse than the pre-treatment malocclusion.

This patient has a severe malocclusion and treatment, if attempted, would involve the use of a functional appliance followed by fixed appliances.

2. What would treatment need to achieve to ensure stability?

As discussed above, stability can only be ensured if the patient has competent lips and the upper incisors are under lower lip control, i.e. the lower lip functions in front of the upper incisors.

Case 3

Orthodontic assessment

This patient has a Class III malocclusion on a Class III skeletal base with maxillary retrognathia and mild mandibular prognathia. The vertical proportions are average and there is facial symmetry. The lips are habitually competent and the naso-labial angle is average.

Intra-orally, the patient is in the late mixed dentition with the LRE retained and UR45 partially erupted. The LLS is well aligned and slightly retroclined; some leeway space remains around LL5. The ULS is mildly crowded in relation to the upper permanent canines and is upright. In occlusion, in the inter-cuspal position (ICP) the overjet is reversed (−2mm) and the overbite is increased and complete.

The buccal segment relationship is Class I on the molars bilaterally and ¼ unit Class III on the canines bilaterally. There are crossbites of UR21 and UL12456. There is a crossbite tendency of UR65. The centre-lines are co-incident with each other and with the facial midline. There is an anterior displacement of the mandible of 2.5mm from an edge-to-edge incisor

relationship in the retruded contact position (RCP).

Problem list

- Patient's complaint: his bite
- Class III skeletal pattern
- Mandibular displacement
- Anterior and posterior crossbites

Answers to questions

1. Would you use a URA to correct the anterior crossbite? Yes, it is appropriate to correct the anterior crossbite with a URA as an interceptive measure.

Rationale: There is currently a marked mandibular displacement from the RCP, which is exacerbating the Class III skeletal pattern and the upper incisors are not already proclined. There is a deep overbite in the displaced position and, therefore, correction of the anterior crossbite could well be stable. Treatment with a URA now may well preclude the necessity for any further orthodontic intervention at a future time, but this will *very much depend* on the amount of mandibular growth that occurs as the patient goes through his adolescent growth spurt. *The patient and parents/guardian should be warned about the possible future effects of mandibular growth.*

Appliance design

A suggested design is shown in Figure 6.18.

2. Would you use a URA to correct the posterior crossbites?

Before deciding whether to correct the posterior crossbites, it will be necessary to assess the transverse relationship in the RCP, as in the ICP (the displaced position) a wider part of the mandibular arch is occluding against a narrower part of the maxillary arch than would be the case in the RCP. Even if a posterior crossbite remains in the RCP, as long as there is no lateral displacement

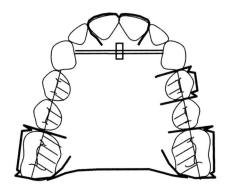

Please construct an upper removable appliance to procline UR2 – UL2:

1. Orthodontic screw in position shown

2. Adams' clasps UR6, UL4, UL6 – 0.7 mm hard ss wire

3. Southend clasp UR1, UL1 – 0.7 mm hard ss wire

4. ½ occlusal coverage posterior capping

5. Baseplate split as shown

Figure 6.18 Laboratory prescription for a URA to procline UR21, UL12 (Case 3).

associated with this, then correction is not required. Indeed, if correction is attempted, which then partially relapses, it is possible to cause a mandibular displacement iatrogenically.

Case 4

Orthodontic assessment

This patient has a mild Class II skeletal pattern with an average or slightly increased FMPA and average lower anterior face height. She has no facial asymmetry and has competent lips.

The patient is in the permanent dentition but has mild gingivitis. She has mild crowding in the lower arch but slightly more severe crowding in the upper arch. The ULS is slightly retroclined but the LLS is normally inclined clinically. UR1 and UR3 are mesio-palatally rotated.

In occlusion, the incisor relationship is a mild Class II division 2; the overbite is slightly increased, but complete to tooth except on UR3. The centre-lines are co-incident (and correct, though this cannot be seen from the photographs). UR3 is in crossbite.

The buccal segment relationships are ½ unit Class II bilaterally. There are no displacements on closure.

Problem list

- Patient's complaint: crooked teeth
- Mild gingivitis
- Mild Class II skeletal pattern
- Crowding in both arches
- Rotated teeth
- Crossbite of UR3
- Reduced overbite on UR3
- ½ unit Class II buccal segment relationships

Answers to questions

1. Suitable for removable appliance treatment to push UR3 over the bite?

   No, this case is not suitable for treatment with a URA to push UR3 over the bite.

Rationale: URAs cannot de-rotate teeth, so the tooth would remain rotated even if correction were attempted.

There is also a slight lack of space and the overbite is reduced. If UR3 were corrected, the overbite would reduce even further and UR3 is very likely to drop back into crossbite. However, the lack of space would prevent movement of UR3.

Fixed appliances would be needed to correct this patient's malocclusion once oral hygiene was sufficiently improved.

Case 5

Orthodontic assessment

This patient has a mild Class II skeletal pattern with average vertical proportions; no facial asymmetry and competent lips. She has an obtuse naso-labial angle.

The patient is in the mixed dentition and has marked, generalised gingivitis. There is also evidence of caries in the deciduous teeth.

The arches are mildly crowded. The ULS and LLS are normally inclined clinically, except for UR2 (retroclined).

In occlusion, the incisor relationship is Class I and the overjet is within normal limits The overbite is average and complete to tooth; the upper centre-line is 1 mm to the right of the facial midline, but the lower is correct (although not visible in the photographs).

The buccal segment relationship is ¼ unit Class II bilaterally. There is a slight forward displacement on closure associated with UR2.

Problem list

- Mother's complaint: crossbite of UR2
- Generalised gingivitis
- Caries
- Mandibular displacement
- Mild crowding in both arches

Answers to questions

1. Suitable for URA treatment to push UR2 over the bite?
   Yes.

Rationale: The patient has a favourable skeletal pattern (i.e. not severe skeletal Class II) and there is a forward displacement on closure (the patient can achieve an edge-to-edge bite of the lower incisors on UR2). The overbite on UR2 is favourable. The inclination of UR2 is also favourable since it is tipped toward the palate and would thus bear tipping forward. However, there is insufficient room to move the tooth forward, but providing due care is taken to ensure the upper canine is not erupting into the path of UR2, space can be made by extraction of both upper deciduous canines once the appliance has been fitted. The URC and ULC

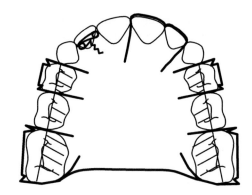

Please construct an upper removable appliance to procline UR2:

1. Z-spring UR2 – 0.5 mm hard ss wire
2. Adams' clasps UR6, UL6 – 0.7 mm hard ss wire
3. Adams' clasps URD, ULD – 0.6 mm hard ss wire
4. Southend clasp UL12 – 0.7 mm hard ss wire
5. ½ occlusal coverage posterior capping UR6 – URD and ULD – UL6

Figure 6.19 Laboratory prescription for a URA to procline UR2 (Case 5).

would need to be extracted to prevent further centre-line discrepancy.

It is important to note that prior to treatment starting, the patient and parent/guardian should be warned that the overjet may increase following correction of UR2, as the displacement is corrected. The mandible may therefore drop back as it no longer has to be brought forward (displaced forward) to 'clear' the instanding UR2.

Appliance design

A suggested design is shown in Figure 6.19.

Case 6

Orthodontic assessment

This patient has a severe Class II division 1 malocclusion on a severe Class II skeletal base due to mandibular retrognathia. The lower anterior face height is reduced, but the FMPA is average. There is facial symmetry. The lips are incompetent with a lower lip trap behind the upper incisor teeth. The naso-labial angle is average.

Intra-orally, the patient is in the permanent dentition with the exception of the previously extracted UR4, LR4 and LL4. UL4 is diminutive. The oral hygiene is good despite some extrinsic staining. A number of the posterior teeth are heavily restored. The LLS is reasonably well aligned and, clinically, normally inclined, but there is marked distal tipping of LR3 and LL3, and an increased curve of Spee. The ULS is irregular, with a mesio-palatal rotation of UR1, and of normal inclination clinically, with marked mesio-buccal rotations of UR5 and UL4.

In occlusion, the overjet is increased (12 mm) and the overbite is increased and complete to the palatal mucosa. The buccal segment relationship on the right is ½ unit Class II on the molars and a full unit Class II on the canines. On the left, the buccal segment relationship is ¼ unit Class II on the molars and 1½ units Class II on the canines. UR5 and UL4 are in scissors bite with the lower teeth. The upper centre-line is 4 mm to the right of the lower centre-line and the facial midline.

Problem list

- Patient's complaint: top teeth stick out
- Severe skeletal Class II
- Reduced vertical dimensions
- Severe rotations of UR5, UR1 and UL4
- Increased overjet (12 mm)
- Increased and complete overbite
- Class II buccal segments, especially canine relationship
- Scissors bite of UR5 and UL4
- Upper centre-line shift to right

Answers to questions

1. Could a URA be used to decrease the overjet after extraction of UL4? No.

2. Could a URA be used to correct the upper centre-line after extraction of the UL4?
   No.

Rationale: The patient has a severe Class II skeletal pattern with a retrognathic mandible and, therefore, the Class II division 1 incisor relationship is not so much due to the position of the upper incisors, but to the mandible being set back. The naso-labial angle is average, with the upper incisors being normally inclined, confirming that the maxilla and upper teeth are in the correct position.

As the upper incisor teeth are normally inclined and the upper centre-line has not shifted to the right due to tipping of the upper incisor teeth, reduction of the overjet and correction of the upper centre-line require bodily movement of the teeth, which can only be achieved with fixed appliances.

Overjet correction will only be stable if the upper incisors are brought under lower lip control. In a case such as this, when the patient has a severe Class II skeletal pattern, reducing the overjet to this extent with a URA would excessively retrocline the upper incisors and turn a Class II division 1 malocclusion into a Class II division 2 malocclusion at the end of treatment. Retroclination of the upper incisors to this extent would also cause the upper lip to drop back, accentuating the nose and causing the lower part of the face to slope backwards from nose to chin, compromising facial aesthetics.

Excessive retroclination of the upper incisors would also occur using fixed appliances in this case, due to the severity of the Class II skeletal pattern and, as the overbite is also very deep, the only sensible treatment approach for this patient would be a combination of fixed appliances and orthognathic surgery.

3. What other aspect of the malocclusion could a URA be used to treat?
   A URA with a flat anterior biteplane could be used initially to reduce the overbite and aid tooth movement with fixed appli-

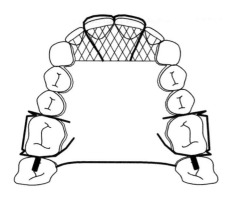

Please construct an upper removable appliance to reduce the overbite:

1. Adams' clasps UR6, UL6 – 0.7 mm hard ss wire

2. Southend clasp UR1, UL1 – 0.7 mm hard ss wire

3. Occlusal rests UR7, UL7 – 0.7 mm hard ss wire

4. Baseplate – please extend posteriorly by 14 mm (OJ 12 mm) and cover 1/2 of the height of the upper central incisor crowns

Figure 6.20 Laboratory prescription for a URA with a FABP to reduce the overbite (Case 6).

ances by unlocking the occlusion. However, this should only be undertaken as part of a comprehensive treatment plan that would also include the use of fixed appliances and orthognathic surgery for optimal results in terms of dental and facial aesthetics.

Appliance design

A suggested design is shown in Figure 6.20.

Case 7

Orthodontic assessment

The patient has a Class I malocclusion on a Class I skeletal base with average vertical proportions and a mild mandibular asymmetry to the left. The lips are habitually competent with an average naso-labial angle.

Intra-orally, the patient is in the mixed dentition with all four first permanent molars and all upper and lower permanent incisor teeth erupted. The oral hygiene requires improvement. The LLS is well aligned and the ULS is mildly spaced. Both upper and lower incisors are normally inclined clinically. There is a small amount of gingival recession labially on LL2.

In the ICP the overjet is average (3 mm) and the overbite is average and complete to tooth. The buccal segment relationship is Class I on the right and ½ unit Class II on the left. There are crossbites affecting UL2–UL6. The upper centre-line is coincident with the facial midline and the lower centre-line is 3 mm to the left of the upper centre-line, but coincident with the chin point. There is a mandibular displacement to the left of 3 mm.

Problem list

- Poor oral hygiene
- Mandibular displacement
- Unilateral posterior crossbite on left
- Anterior crossbite of UL2
- Lower centre-line shift to left

Answers to questions

1. Would you use a URA to correct the posterior crossbite and/or UL2 position? Yes. In this case, assuming oral hygiene can be improved, it is appropriate to use a URA as an interceptive measure to correct the position of UL2 and the crossbite.

Rationale: The reasons for doing this are to prevent any further deterioration in the gingival condition of LL2, as the recession is being caused by UL2 being in crossbite with LL2. Also, when there is a significant lateral mandibular displacement, as here, it is sensible to eliminate the displacement before all the permanent teeth erupt to discourage asymmetric growth of the mandible and to encourage the permanent teeth to erupt into the appropriate positions.

Appliance design

A suggested design is shown in Figure 6.21.

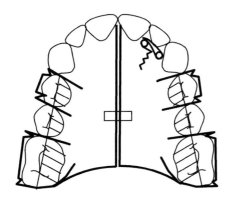

Please construct an upper removable appliance to expand the upper arch and move UL2 labially:

1. Midline expansion screw

2. Z-spring UL2 – 0.5 mm hard ss wire

3. Adams' clasps UR6, UL6 – 0.7 mm hard ss wire

4. Adams' clasps URD, ULD – 0.6 mm hard ss wire

5. ½ occlusal coverage posterior capping

6. Midline split in baseplate as indicated

Figure 6.21 Laboratory prescription for a URA to procline UL2 and correct the posterior crossbite by expansion of the upper arch (Case 7).

Case 8

Orthodontic assessment

This patient has a mild Class III skeletal pattern with average vertical proportions; his chin is slightly to the right and he has competent lips.

The patient is in the early mixed dentition and has good oral hygiene. Currently there is no crowding in either arch. Clinically, the LLS is slightly proclined and the ULS is normally inclined. However, UR1 is mesio-palatally rotated.

In occlusion, the incisor relationship is Class III and the overjet is 1 mm on the upper left incisors but –1 mm on the upper right incisors. The overbite is reduced but complete to tooth, whilst the upper centre-line is correct but the lower is to the right.

The buccal segment relationship is Class I on the right and ½ unit Class II on the left; there is a crossbite on the URC and URD, whilst on the left there is a crossbite affecting ULCDE6. Anteriorly only the upper right central and lateral incisors are in crossbite. However, there was a displacement both forward and to the right on closure.

Problem list

- Parents' complaint: crooked teeth and teeth biting the wrong way round
- Skeletal Class III pattern (hence risk of unfavourable growth)
- Displacement on closure
- Class III incisor relationship with UR1 and UR2 in crossbite
- UR1 rotated
- Reduced overbite
- Bilateral crossbites

Answers to questions

1. Suitable for URA treatment to push the upper right central and lateral incisor over the bite?

   No, this patient is not ideally suited.

Rationale: This patient has a reduced overbite. Therefore, if the incisors were pushed over the bite, the overbite will reduce even further, resulting in questionable stability.

In addition, UR1 is rotated and removable appliances are unable to de-rotate teeth.

Since the patient has a forward displacement on closure and the incisal inclinations are reasonably favourable, an experienced clinician might consider an attempt at correction (in order to provide more space for the unerupted dentition), given that two of the incisors are over the bite. However, if attempted, the patient and parent/guardian should be strongly warned of the risk of relapse. The rotation would have to be accepted.

Case 9

Orthodontic assessment

The patient has a mild Class III malocclusion on a very mild Class II skeletal pattern with average vertical proportions and a mild mandibular asymmetry to the left. The lips are habitually competent and the naso-labial angle is average.

Intra-orally, the patient is in the mixed dentition with the four first permanent molars and the upper and lower permanent incisor teeth erupted. Both the ULS and LLS are spaced. Clinically, the lower incisors are slightly reclined and the upper incisors are normally inclined, but UR1 is positioned more labial and more gingival than the other incisors.

In occlusion, the overjet is slightly reduced (2 mm) to UL1 and the overbite is reduced and complete to tooth.

The buccal segment relationship is Class I bilaterally. There are no crossbites. The upper centre-line is coincident with the facial midline and the lower centre-line is 3 mm to the left of the upper centre-line.

Problem list

- Patient's complaint: appearance of UR1
- Position of UR1
- Lower centre-line shift to the left

Answers to questions

1. Could a URA be used to bring UR1 down into a more ideal position? Yes, interceptive treatment with a URA to align UR1 is appropriate.

Rationale: Not only will alignment of UR1 improve the aesthetics, but it will prevent UR2 from drifting mesially, palatal to UR1, which would reduce the space available for UR1 to be aligned in the future.

Appliance design

A suggested design is shown in Figure 6.22.

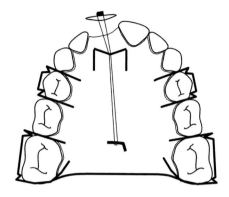

Please construct an upper removable appliance to allow extrusion of UR1:

1. "Goalpost" positioned behind upper incisors – pt has a 3 mm overjet and an average overbite

2. Hook positioned in baseplate opposite first permanent molars, facing distally

3. Adams' clasps UR6, UL6 – 0.7 mm hard ss wire

4. Adams' clasps URD, ULD – 0.6 mm hard ss wire

5. Baseplate

Figure 6.22   Laboratory prescription for a URA to extrude UR1 (Case 9).

Case 10

Orthodontic assessment

This patient has a mild Class II skeletal pattern with slightly increased vertical proportions; her chin point is slightly to the right. She has habitually competent lips and a slightly obtuse naso-labial angle.

The patient is in the mixed dentition and now has good oral health and dental health following oral hygiene instruction.

The lower arch is normally inclined clinically, but also mildly crowded. The upper arch is well aligned and of normal inclination, but UL1 is unerupted; there is an erupted supernumerary in the UL1 position and the ULB is retained. Assuming the upper laterals are present, they will be severely crowded when they erupt.

In occlusion, the incisor relationship is mildly Class III and the overjet is reduced (1 mm), as is the overbite which is complete to tooth. The lower centre-line is 1 mm to the right, but the upper is correct.

The buccal segment relationship is ½ unit Class II on the right, but Class I on the left. There is also a slight, right-sided, unilateral crossbite and, although this is associated with a slight displacement on closure, it is largely related to the exfoliating LRC.

Problem list

- Patient's complaint: appearance of top front teeth
- Erupted supernumerary and retained ULB
- Insufficient space for UL1
- Centre-line discrepancy
- Potential crowding in both arches, especially U2s
- Reduced overjet and overbite
- Crossbite on right side

The cause of this patient's malocclusion is the presence of the supernumerary, which is blocking the eruption of UL1 and UL2. This type of supernumerary is known as a mesiodens or conical supernumerary.

Answers to questions

1. Patient suitable for treatment using a URA?
    Yes. However, treatment will be aimed at maintaining space once the obstruction to the eruption of UL1 has been removed and sufficient space has been created.

Rationale: The patient's skeletal pattern and extra-oral features are not particularly relevant in this case at this time as the aim of treatment at this stage is purely getting UL1 into its normal position. This may require more than one stage of treatment. However, as this is a timely referral, there is a good chance that UL1 will erupt (if the root apex has not yet closed) without requiring orthodontic extrusion with

aspects of fixed appliance intervention. Of course, depending on how the other teeth erupt and how the patient grows, other treatment may be required at a later stage. The patient and parent/guardian should be advised of this prior to treatment starting.

A space-maintaining URA would need to be designed and fitted. Assessment of all relevant records suggests that removal of the UL$ and ULB would provide sufficient space for UL1 to erupt. The appliance would need to be worn for a period of at least 6 months and frequently much longer, but the time required will of course be affected by the position of UL1. Radiographic investigation would be needed to assess the progress of UL1 if it is not showing obvious clinical signs of erupting during this time. If significant progress is not clear within 9–12 months of the supernumerary being removed, surgical exposure may then be needed to allow active, orthodontic extrusion of UL1.

Appliance design

A suggested design is shown in Figure 6.23.

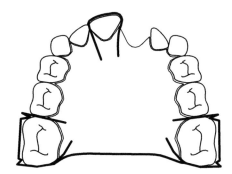

Please construct an upper removable appliance to maintain the space for the unerupted UL1:

1. Adams' clasps UR6, UL6 – 0.7 mm hard ss wire

2. Southend clasp UR1 – 0.6 mm

3. Baseplate with well-fitting colleting

Figure 6.23 Laboratory prescription for a URA to maintain the space for the eruption of UL1 (Case 10).

Case 11

Orthodontic assessment

This patient has a Class I (tending towards very mild Class III) skeletal pattern with an average lower anterior face height, but slightly increased FMPA. There is facial symmetry, but mildly incompetent lips.

The patient is in the permanent dentition and has mild, generalised gingivitis. She has mild crowding in the lower arch, but much more severe crowding in the upper arch.

The LLS is somewhat retroclined clinically, although the ULS is normally inclined. The upper canines are totally buccally excluded and are distally angulated. The upper laterals are almost in contact with the first premolars.

In occlusion, the incisor relationship is Class III and the overjet is edge-to-edge. The overbite is also edge-to-edge whilst the centre-lines are co-incident and correct.

The buccal segment relationship is ¼ unit Class II on the right and ½ unit Class II on the left; there are crossbite tendencies bilaterally in both buccal segments, but only the upper lateral incisors are in crossbite. However, there are no displacements on closure.

Problem list

* Oral hygiene
* Patient's complaint: crooked teeth
* Tendency towards skeletal Class III pattern
* Slightly increased vertical proportions
* Risk of unfavourable growth
* Crowding in both arches with buccally excluded and distally angulated upper canines
* Retroclined LLS
* Class III incisor relationship
* No overbite but crossbite of the upper lateral incisors

Answers to questions

Suitable for URA treatment:

1. To allow spontaneous alignment of both the upper canines following loss of both upper first premolars?
2. To align the buccally crowded canines following upper first premolar extractions?
3. To correct the upper lateral incisor crossbite?

No, a URA is not suitable for correcting any aspect of the malocclusion.

Rationale: Dentally, this patient is relatively mature as she is no longer in the mixed dentition and the upper canines are well erupted and distally angulated. Therefore, if the patient were fitted with a space maintainer and the upper first premolars extracted, it is highly unlikely that the upper canines would show much spontaneous movement. Remember that teeth tend to tip towards extraction spaces, so if they are already distally tipped, then they will tend to tip even more distally. This would not be favourable and would have virtually no effect on space closure. In fact, the patient would be worse off than if nothing had been done, since they would still have the crowding but now combined with large extraction spaces. Even if they were mesially angulated, given the dental maturity of the patient, spontaneous alignment at this age would be very limited.

The problem regarding the use of a URA to align the buccally crowded canines following loss of the upper first premolars is that this patient has distally angulated upper canines. Palatal finger springs would be contraindicated as the canines are buccal. However, more importantly, the distal angulation means tipping is contraindicated too, since URAs will cause the upper canines to become even more grossly distally tipped. This would result in a very poor contact and poor appearance. Furthermore, depending on the space available relative to the width of the canines, there may not be enough space.

Regarding the use of a URA to correct the upper lateral incisor crossbite, this patient has no overbite. Therefore if the upper laterals were pushed over the bite they would relapse.

The patient may yet also grow unfavourably. Furthermore, there is insufficient space as the upper canines would be in the way.

The patient's oral health is too poor to consider any immediate orthodontic intervention. If any treatment with fixed appliances is to be undertaken for this patient, she would need to improve her oral hygiene first. In view of the Class III tendency, treatment may, at this stage, be limited to the upper arch only.

Case 12

Orthodontic assessment

The patient has a Class I malocclusion on a mild Class II skeletal base with average vertical proportions and facial symmetry. The lips are habitually competent and the naso-labial angle is average.

Intra-orally, the patient is in the mixed dentition with all four first permanent molars and the four lower permanent incisors erupted. The LLS is slightly irregular and spaced. In the upper arch, UR2, UL1 and UL2 are erupted, but UR1 is unerupted and is visible under the gingivae in the labial sulcus. UR2 and UL1 have moved mesially to take up some of the space available for UR1 to erupt and UR2 is mesially tipped.

In occlusion, the overjet is average and the overbite is average and complete to tooth. The buccal segment relationship is Class I bilaterally. There are no crossbites. The upper centre-line is slightly to the right of the lower centre-line and of the facial midline.

Problem list

- Unerupted UR1
- Insufficient space for UR1 to erupt

Answers to questions

1. Would you use a URA to re-create the space for UR1 to erupt? Yes, it is appropriate to use a URA as an interceptive measure to re-

create the space so that UR1 may erupt. However, it is essential to investigate why UR1 has not erupted, so that the appropriate intervention may be taken to ensure that it can erupt once the space has been re-created. In this case, unusually, UR1 was ectopically positioned, but was otherwise normal.

Appliance design

A suggested design is shown in Figure 6.24.

2. Would you advocate the removal of any teeth prior to activating any appliance you might use?

    In some cases where space is to be re-opened for an unerupted incisor, then it is necessary to create space into which to retract the lateral incisors by removal of the primary canine teeth. However, this would only be indicated in cases where the buccal

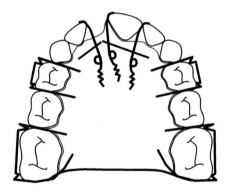

Please construct an upper removable appliance to retract (distalise) UR2, UL1 and UL2 to re-open space for UR1:

1. Palatal finger springs UR2, UL1 and UL2 – 0.5 mm hard ss wire with box and guard wire

2. Adams' clasps UR6, UL6 – 0.7 mm hard ss wire

3. Adams' clasps URD, ULD – 0.6 mm hard ss wire

4. Baseplate saddled as indicated

Figure 6.24 Laboratory prescription for a URA to recreate the space for the eruption of UR1 by distalising UR2, UL1 and UL2 (Case 12).

segment relationship was Class II. In a case like this, where the buccal segments are a well–inter-digitated Class I and the LLS is slightly spaced, then it should be possible to re-create enough space for the eruption of UR1 without extracting teeth.

When it is necessary to extract the primary canine teeth, the patient and parent should be warned that the original crowding of the permanent teeth will be moved to the position of the permanent canine teeth.

Case 13

Orthodontic assessment

The patient has a Class III incisor relationship on a severe Class III skeletal base due to maxillary hypoplasia. He has a reduced lower anterior face height and an average FMPA. The mandible is symmetrical. His lips are competent with an obtuse naso-labial angle.

Intra-orally, he is in the permanent dentition and, although the upper permanent canine teeth are unerupted and palpable buccally, they are short of space to erupt. The lower right first permanent molar has been previously extracted. Oral hygiene is very poor. There is mild irregularity of the LLS, which is retroclined. The ULS is proclined and spaced currently, but it is potentially severely crowded due to the upper canines being unerupted.

In occlusion, the overjet is reversed (−2 mm) and the overbite is increased and complete. The buccal segment relationship is a full unit Class III on the left and a ½ unit Class III on the right. The upper centre-line is to the right of the lower centre-line and the facial midline. All the upper teeth apart from UL6 are in crossbite with the lower teeth. There is no mandibular displacement on closure.

Problem list

- Poor oral health (risk of demineralisation)
- Severe Class III skeletal pattern (unfavourable growth)

- Severe crowding in the upper arch with impacted upper canines
- LLS already retroclined
- ULS already proclined
- Transverse discrepancy with all upper teeth, except for UL6, being in crossbite with lower teeth, and the upper teeth are already flared buccally
- Upper centre-line shift to the right

Answers to questions

1. Assuming that oral hygiene improves to the required standard, could a URA be used to correct the anterior crossbite? No.

Rationale: The anterior crossbite is due to the severe Class III skeletal discrepancy and the patient cannot achieve an edge-to-edge incisor relationship. Furthermore, the patient has outgrown the previous correction and there has already been significant dento-alveolar compensation for the skeletal pattern, partly due to the previous URA treatment. The upper incisors are very proclined and correction of the anterior crossbite by further proclination may cause non-axial loading on the upper incisors, which compromises the supporting tissues and may lead to root resorption. Very proclined upper incisors are also very unaesthetic in appearance. Furthermore, as the patient is only 11 years old and has yet to go through his adolescent growth spurt, the Class III skeletal pattern is likely to get worse. In all cases where the upper canines are unerupted, it is essential to ensure that any movement of the lateral incisor is not going to tip the root of this tooth into the crown of the canine, so running the risk of root resorption.

2. Would you use a URA to hold open the space for the unerupted upper permanent canine teeth following extraction of the upper first premolar teeth?

A URA could be used as a space maintainer to allow the eruption of the upper permanent canine teeth after the removal of the upper first premolars. *However,* this would either be as part of a more involved treatment plan involving full correction of his malocclusion, *or* part of a compromise plan.

Rationale: Full correction would entail fixed appliances and orthognathic surgery, and would take place at a later date towards the very end of growth. Alternatively, a compromise plan, which would not aim to correct any other aspect of the malocclusion apart from creating space for the permanent canine teeth to erupt, could be undertaken earlier.

Appliance design

A suggested design is shown in Figure 6.25.

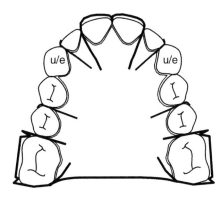

Please construct an upper removable appliance to maintain the space for the unerupted upper canine teeth following the extraction of the upper first premolars:

1. Adams' clasps UR6, UL6 – 0.7 mm hard ss wire

2. Southend clasp UR1, UL1 – 0.7 mm hard ss wire

3. Stops distal to UR2, UL2 and mesial to UR5, UL5 – 0.6 mm hard ss wire

4. Baseplate with well-adapted colleting

Figure 6.25 Laboratory prescription for a URA maintain the space for the eruption of the upper permanent canine teeth following the extraction of the upper first premolars (Case 13).

3. Could a URA be used to correct the posterior crossbites? No.

Rationale: The transverse discrepancy is due to the severe Class III antero-posterior skeletal pattern rather than to a narrowing of the maxillary arch *per se.* As both upper and lower arches are wider in the molar regions than in the canine regions, a severe Class III pattern leads to a wider part of the lower arch being in occlusion with a narrower part of the upper arch, creating the crossbite. URAs can only tip teeth. The upper buccal segments are already very tipped in a buccal direction. Any further tipping would lead to them being taken out of occlusion with the lower teeth or only the palatal cusps would be in occlusion. This reduces the ability to produce a well–inter-digitated occlusion at the end of treatment, leading to relapse of the upper arch expansion, with the potential to cause occlusal interferences and, hence, a mandibular displacement that the patient does not have currently.

4. Could a URA be used to correct the upper centre-line shift? No.

Rationale: Correction of the upper centre-line shift requires bodily movement of the upper incisor teeth. URAs are only able to tip teeth. If a URA were used, the crowns could be tipped into a better position, but the root position would only change minimally, creating a very unaesthetic tipped appearance of the upper incisor teeth.

Case 14

Orthodontic assessment

This patient has a mild Class II skeletal pattern with average or only slightly increased vertical proportions; there is no facial asymmetry and incompetent lips.

The patient is in the mixed dentition and has good oral hygiene and dental health generally, although the LLE is heavily restored.

The lower arch is very mildly crowded and the upper arch is well aligned, except for the retroclined UR1 and retained and discoloured UR A which is firm. The ULS and LLS are normally inclined clinically, except for UR1 (retroclined).

In occlusion, the incisor relationship is Class I and the overjet is within normal limits. The overbite is slightly increased and complete to tooth; the centre-lines are co-incident and correct.

The buccal segment relationship is ½ unit Class II bilaterally. There is a slight forward displacement on closure associated with UR1.

Problem list

- Patient's complaint: top teeth not showing
- UR A retained, non-vital and firm
- UR1 in crossbite
- Forward displacement on UR1
- Very mild crowding in the lower arch

Answers to questions

1. What is the cause of this patient's malocclusion and is the patient suitable for correction of the UR1 crossbite using a URA?
   The cause of this patient's malocclusion is the non-vital UR A. This probably became non-vital following an episode of trauma when the patient was younger and the tooth becoming ankylosed. Due to its failure to shed normally, this has resulted in UR1 being deflected into crossbite.

   Yes, this patient is suitable for URA treatment to push UR1 over the bite.

Rationale: The patient has a favourable skeletal pattern (i.e. not severe skeletal Class II) and there is a forward displacement on closure (patient can make edge-to-edge bite of the lower incisors on UR1). The overbite on UR1 is favourable. The inclination of UR1 is also favourable, since it is tipped toward the palate and would thus bear tipping forward. There is sufficient room to move the tooth forwards, providing the UR A is extracted once the appliance has been fitted.

It is important to note that prior to treatment starting, the patient and parent/guardian

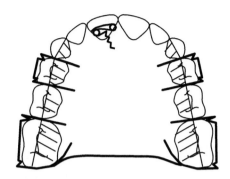

Please construct an upper removable appliance to procline UR1:

1. Z spring UR1 – 0.5 mm hard ss wire

2. Adams' clasps UR6, UL6 – 0.7 mm hard ss wire

3. Adams' clasps URD, ULD – 0.6 mm hard ss wire

4. ½ occlusal coverage posterior capping UR6 – URC and ULC – UL6

Figure 6.26 Laboratory prescription for a URA to procline UR1 (Case 14).

should be warned that the overjet may increase following correction of UR1 as the displacement is corrected. The mandible may therefore drop back as it no longer has to be brought forward (displaced forward) to 'clear' the instanding UR1.

It is possible that if the UR A had been extracted when UR1 started to erupt, the problem could have been avoided.

Incidentally, the crowding in the lower arch is too mild to warrant any treatment.

Appliance design

A suggested design is shown in Figure 6.26.

Case 15

Orthodontic assessment

This patient has a severe Class II division 1 malocclusion on a moderate Class II skeletal base with average vertical proportions and facial symmetry. The lips are incompetent with a lower lip trap behind the upper incisors and the naso-labial angle is obtuse.

Intra-orally, the patient is in the permanent dentition with the exception of unerupted LL5. UL5 is partially erupted. The oral health requires a little improvement. The LLS is well aligned and slightly proclined, and the ULS is proclined and spaced, but the upper canines are distally angulated.

In occlusion, the overjet is increased (12 mm), the overbite is average and complete to palatal mucosa, and the buccal segment relationship is ¾ unit Class II bilaterally. There are no crossbites and the upper and lower centre-lines are co-incident with each other and with the facial midline.

Problem list

- Oral hygiene
- Patient's complaint: top teeth stick out
- Moderate skeletal Class II
- Grossly incompetent lips and lower lip trap
- Increased overjet
- Class II buccal segment relationship

Answers to questions

1. Could this patient be treated by extraction of upper first premolars and URA(s) to retract the upper canines and then reduce the overjet? No.

Rationale: The patient has a moderate Class II skeletal pattern with a retrognathic mandible and, therefore, the Class II division 1 incisor relationship is not so much due to the position of the upper incisors, but more to the mandible being set back. The proclination of the upper incisors is caused by the lower lip trap. The naso-labial angle is obtuse.

As URAs are only able to tip teeth and as the upper canine teeth are already distally angulated, retracting the upper canines into the space created by extraction of the upper first premolars would cause them to become even more distally tipped, as they would need to be retracted by the whole width of a premolar (7 mm). Distally angulated canines are unaesthetic and tipping a tooth to this extent is prone to relapse, which would lead to re-opening of the extraction space and an increase in overjet.

Although the upper incisors are proclined pre-treatment, overjet correction will only be stable if the upper incisors are brought under lower lip control. Reducing the overjet to this extent with a URA would excessively retrocline the upper incisors and turn a Class II division 1 malocclusion into a Class II division 2 malocclusion with a potentially traumatic overbite.

Treatment for this patient's severe malocclusion would involve a functional appliance followed by fixed appliances.

Case 16

Orthodontic assessment

The patient has a Class III incisor relationship on a mild Class III skeletal base with maxillary retrognathia. The lower anterior face height is reduced with an average FMPA. There is a mandibular asymmetry to the right. The lips are competent and the naso-labial angle is obtuse.

Intra-orally, the patient is in the permanent dentition with marked gingival recession labially on both the lower central incisors. The LLS is mildly crowded and normally inclined clinically and the ULS is irregular, with the upper central incisors slightly retroclined clinically.

In the ICP the overjet to UR1 is reversed (−1 mm) and the overbite is slightly reduced and complete to tooth. The buccal segment relationship is ¼ unit Class III on the right and ½ unit Class III on the left. UR1 and UL1 are in crossbite with LR1 and LL1, and UL2 is in crossbite with LL3. The lower centre-line is to the right of the facial midline and to the right of the upper centre-line by 2.5 mm. There is a mandibular displacement from an edge-to-edge incisor relationship in the RCP, anteriorly and to the right in the ICP.

Problem list

- Patient's complaint: position of front teeth
- Class III skeletal pattern
- Mandibular asymmetry
- Mandibular displacement anteriorly and to the right, exacerbating the Class III skeletal pattern and the mandibular asymmetry
- Gingival recession of LR1 and LL1
- Anterior crossbite in the ICP
- Slightly reduced overbite

Answers to questions

1. Would you use a URA to correct the position of the upper central incisors? Yes, it is appropriate to use a URA as an interceptive measure in this case.

Rationale: Correcting the anterior crossbite may help protect the supporting tissues of the lower central incisors and improve aesthetics. Using a simple treatment now will allow further assessment of mandibular growth as the patient goes through her adolescent growth spurt prior to determining a definitive treatment plan.

Although the overbite is slightly reduced, the use of posterior capping will help increase the overbite slightly and, as only a small amount of proclination of the upper central incisors is required to eliminate the mandibular displacement and, hence, the anterior crossbite, the overbite should be sufficient to maintain the correction.

It is important to note that prior to treatment starting, the patient and parent/guardian should be advised that the overjet will increase following correction of UR1 and UL1 as the displacement is corrected. The mandible may therefore drop back as it no longer has to be brought forward (displaced forward) to 'clear' the instanding upper incisors. However, in a Class III case this is not likely to be a problem. In addition, the UL2 which is in crossbite and has minimal overbite and is also rotated, would have to be accepted at this time.

Appliance design
A suggested design is shown in Figure 6.27.

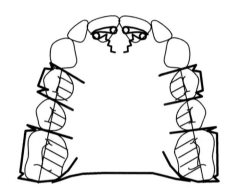

Please construct an upper removable appliance to procline UR1, UL1:

1. Z spring UR1, UL1 – 0.5 mm hard ss wire

2. Adams' clasps UR6, UR4, UL4, UL6 – 0.7 mm hard ss wire

3. ½ occlusal coverage posterior capping

Figure 6.27 Laboratory prescription for a URA to procline UR1 and UL1 (Case 16).

Retainers

Retention is the period following active treatment when teeth need to be maintained in their new positions. In most cases, if this phase of treatment does not occur, then there is a very strong chance of relapse. This is because both bone and soft tissues take time to adapt and re-establish their pre-treatment strength.

- Explain some advantages and disadvantages of different types of retainer
- Describe the role of the general dental practitioner in monitoring retainers
- Describe some problems that may occur with retainers
- Understand the need to liaise with the specialist

Learning outcomes

At the end of this chapter you should be able to:

- Explain what relapse is
- Explain the difference between relapse and maturational (or age) changes
- Understand which types of tooth movement/ situations are prone to relapse
- Explain what the purpose of retention and retainers is
- Explain what retention regimes are
- Explain the need for retention with regard to interceptive treatment

What is relapse?

Consider the bone remodelling cycle: the whole cycle takes about 6 months to complete and, since when teeth are moved, bone has to be resorbed (ahead of the root) and deposited (behind the root), the whole bone remodelling cycle applies. Therefore, in order for there to be any prospect of avoiding relapse, retention needs to be for a period of at least 6 months. However, soft tissues obviously also have a role to play, and their adaptability and turnover also influence the likelihood of stability (or the lack of it).

Orthodontic Retainers and Removable Appliances: Principles of Design and Use, First Edition.
Friedy Luther and Zararna Nelson-Moon.
© 2013 Friedy Luther and Zararna Nelson-Moon. Published 2013 by Blackwell Publishing Ltd.

Depending on the location, some or all of the following soft tissues may have a role to play with regard to relapse and stability: the gingivae; periodontal ligament; lips, cheeks and tongue. For all situations however, the gingivae and periodontal ligament will always have a role to play, and adaptation, particularly in the supracrestal gingival (elastic) fibres, will actually take longer than for bone. Indeed, whilst it is thought that these fibres take at least 9 months to re-adapt, it is not certain that these fibres will ever adapt fully to the new tooth positions. This means that there are a number of situations where stability will never really be possible and relapse is a strong possibility.

Many people – dentists included – will tend to term *any* post-active-treatment tooth movement as 'relapse', but this is not strictly true. Furthermore, it is important to be clear about what we actually mean by relapse, as it influences what both operators and patients can expect from treatment. Relapse should be distinguished from maturational or age changes with which it is frequently confused.

Technically and practically, relapse actually means that teeth return either to their pre-treatment position or toward this position.

Features of relapse

- Usually occurs rapidly – within a few weeks or months.
- Often due to operator factors such as incorrect treatment mechanics, e.g. reducing an overjet by proclination of the lower incisors; correcting an incisor crossbite without ensuring there is sufficient overbite to keep the incisor corrected. Such problems may themselves be due to incorrect diagnosis in the first place.
- Occasionally patient factors may be the underlying problem, e.g. the patient fails to wear the retainer either at all or as requested.
- There are situations (noted below) that are prone to relapse *unless* they are 'permanently' retained.

What are maturational changes? How do they differ from relapse?

Several long-term studies have followed up untreated individuals for many years. These studies have demonstrated that teeth tend to move throughout life.

Features of maturational change

Common findings are:

- Inter-canine width reduces with age (more in females than males).
- Crowding tends to increase with age – this is particularly common in the lower incisor region, but other teeth, including the upper incisors, can also be affected.
- Inter-molar width however shows little change.
- Usually occurs slowly – over months or years.
- Occurs in young adults as well as older individuals.
- Can occur even in individuals who have had 'straight teeth' for years.
- Wisdom teeth have frequently been blamed for late lower incisor crowding, but we now know that this occurs regardless of the presence or absence of third molars.

Although other changes may also occur, such as changes in overjet or overbite, the biggest problem is that we cannot yet predict which patients will be most likely to experience such changes.

What is the importance of distinguishing relapse from maturational change?

The crucial point is that orthodontic treatment does not stop teeth moving throughout life; whether treatment involves extractions or not makes no difference. Teeth are not fixed in stone throughout life just because of orthodontic treatment. Therefore, this needs to be explained to all patients about to embark on treatment. Whilst retainers can help reduce the amount of relapse as the bone and soft tissues re-adapt, it is, practically-speaking, impossible to guarantee to any patient that *their teeth will never move from the post-treatment position – even if they continue to wear retainers*. There are several reasons for this:

- Retainers (whether removable or fixed) may break and, as a consequence, the position of the teeth will not be adequately controlled until the retainer can be repaired or a replacement can be fitted. The literature shows that fixed retainers, in particular, have high failure rates.
- Removable retainers may not always be worn as instructed and/or they may be lost.
- Clinicians may not instruct patients adequately.
- With time and use, wires tend to stretch or suffer a reduction in stiffness. Therefore, even when bonded retainers remain attached to the teeth and there is no obvious failure of any of the components, subtle changes may occur, including small spaces opening between teeth and changes in inclination of individual teeth. These have been infrequently documented in the literature to date, but this itself is probably due to the lack of long-term follow-up of patients. Furthermore, it is only comparatively recently that increasing numbers of patients are wearing retainers.

It is often assumed that bonded retainers are more effective than removable retainers. However, as noted above, this is not borne out by studies undertaken so far.

Cases that are particularly prone to relapse and why

There are several situations that are known to be especially prone to relapse:

- Rotations
- Spacing due to small and/or developmentally absent teeth; midline diastemas
- Movements involving significant expansion
- Periodontally involved teeth.

Rotations

In the case of rotations, the issue of relapse relates directly to the soft-tissue factors noted previously. When a tooth is de-rotated, i.e. 'untwisted', the supracrestal gingival (elastic) fibres seem very slow to re-adapt to the new position and indeed may never adapt fully to the new tooth positions. Any residual tension in the gingival fibres is more likely to lead to some degree of relapse, even following many months of retention.

In order to reduce this tendency, a minor surgical procedure known as 'pericision' or 'supracrestal fiberotomy' has been devised. This procedure can be undertaken under local anaesthesia and involves the insertion of a thin scalpel blade down the gingival crevice (until it contacts the alveolus) and circling the blade around the neck of the tooth. The aim is to cut the gingival fibres that insert into the neck of the tooth above the alveolar bone crest, to encourage them to re-adapt to the new tooth position. However, even though this is a simple procedure to undertake, it needs to be done carefully in order to avoid causing any periodontal problems such as recession. Pericision is not really suitable for use in the lower labial segment (LLS) as the teeth are much narrower than in the upper labial segment (ULS), and so too is the gingival cuff. There is therefore a greater risk of iatrogenic periodontal damage.

Nevertheless, even if a patient agrees to pericision being performed, studies suggest that rotational relapse will still not be eliminated and relapse in the region of 20% can be expected. Also, some patients may find the idea of a surgical procedure off-putting.

Spacing due to small and/or developmentally absent teeth: diastemas

Here again, lack of soft-tissue adaptation is the problem. Whilst it may be possible and, indeed, quite straightforward (using fixed appliances) to close spaces of 1–2 mm, the far bigger problem is maintaining space closure. The problem seems to be even greater when attempts are made to close larger spaces. Any break in retainer wear can lead to rapid relapse even when fixed, i.e. bonded, retainers are used.

Maintaining spaces that have been increased for the placement of fixed prostheses, where teeth are developmentally missing in hypodontia cases, is an equally difficult problem. Figure 7.1 shows an example of significant relapse following orthodontic treatment for hypodontia.

In order to help with midline diastema closure, frenectomy has been suggested and performed. However, whilst this may help in some patients, the difficulty is that there is no reliable means of predicting which diastemas are caused by a 'fleshy frenum' and which are not. Alleged signs that a frenectomy may be indicated include: blanching of the incisive papilla when the frenum is stretched by pulling the upper lip forward, or a notch of the alveolus between the upper central incisors visible on an upper anterior occlusal radiograph. Unfortunately, neither of these signs is reliable

enough to be clinically valid. Furthermore, it has been found that with time/age, diastemas tend to reduce spontaneously. The same cannot be said of spaces or spacing due to hypodontia; these spaces have no relationship to frenal attachments.

Movements involving significant expansion

Some expansion can be acceptable. However, relapse occurs when teeth are tipped beyond the basal bone because this causes the teeth to flare outward and, as a consequence, there is little or no occlusal inter-digitation. Likewise, relapse is also inevitable when a crossbite of skeletal aetiology is corrected by tooth movement only. The problems of relapse in these situations are due to a combination of bone, soft-tissue and dental factors.

Periodontally involved teeth

Patients who experience severe periodontal disease lose bone and soft tissue from around the teeth affected. This means that the soft tissue balance is now altered: the pressures from the tongue and lips/cheeks are now less opposed than previously due to the loss of hard and soft periodontal tissues. Consequently, the teeth tend to drift to a new position of balance. However, due to the increased bone and tissue

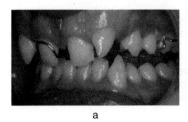 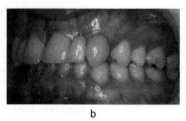 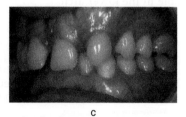

a   b   c

Figure 7.1 Example of the strong relapse tendency of spacing – in this case associated with hypodontia. This patient underwent 2 years of fixed appliance treatment (plus a biteplane) to reduce the spaces between the centrals and open spaces for the upper laterals (a). Bonded bridges were placed (b), but unfortunately, during an hospital admission, one bridge was knocked out by an anaesthetist and within a few days UL3 had slipped forward again and UR1 and UL1 had moved apart (c). The patient had to undergo re-treatment.

turnover (as a result of ongoing disease), a balance is not achieved and the teeth can continue to drift. In addition, tissue pressures from the periodontal ligaments are reduced due to the loss of ligament as a result of disease.

If at some stage the periodontal disease is fully controlled and the patient undergoes orthodontic treatment to re-align the teeth, the result will always be highly unstable. This is because the imbalance between hard and soft tissues around the teeth versus those around the rest of the oral cavity will always remain, as bone and soft tissue cannot be replaced. This leads to constant instability without indefinite retention.

Types of retainers

Currently the choice of retainers divides into removable or fixed retainers. They can be made for either upper or lower arches (or both of course, as is mostly the case) and it is perfectly possible and reasonable that on occasion the two types may be used in the same patient. In contrast to (active) lower removable appliances (LRAs; which generally do not work well in the lower arch), removable retainers generally work perfectly well in the lower arch. This is because these are passive appliances; therefore, there is far less likelihood of the appliance being dislodged since there are no active forces. Active forces often lead to frequent LRA dislodgement due to the much poorer retention being available in the lower arch.

Removable retainers

Two main types of removable retainer exist: Hawley-type (or variations thereof) (Figure 7.2) and vacuum-formed retainers (VFRs; Figure 7.3).

Hawley-type retainers

Manufacture
* All involve an acrylic baseplate with wire-work adapted in custom-fashion to the teeth.

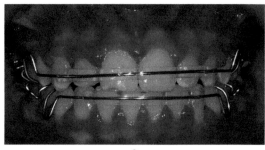

a

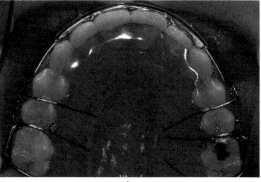

b

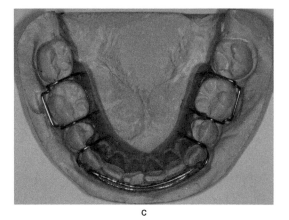

c

Figure 7.2 Examples (a–c) of upper and lower Hawley retainers (modified in these examples with an acrylic facing added to the labial bow to provide extra retention).

* Both the acrylic and wire-work components require direct, hands-on manufacture by a technician to a plaster working model of the patient's own teeth.

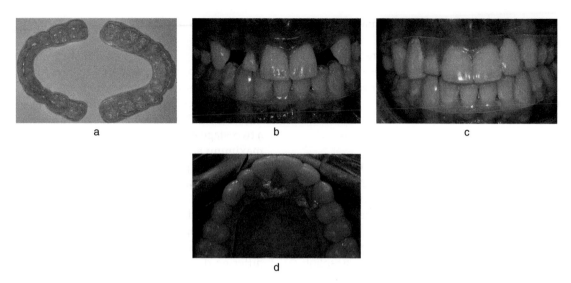

Figure 7.3 Examples of standard upper and lower vacuum-formed retainers (VFRs) (a). (b–d) The VFR has been modified to replace missing teeth.

- They are therefore more expensive and time consuming to make than the vacuum-formed variety.

Advantages

- Do not cover the occlusal surfaces of the teeth. Therefore, following active treatment, if further 'settling in' of the occlusion is required (vertical movements of the upper and lower buccal segments toward each other), this type of retainer can allow this more satisfactorily than the vacuum-formed type.
- Can be used successfully for retaining overjet reduction as they act like a strap across the front of the upper incisors.
- Can be worn whilst eating. This is useful if, for example, an upper Hawley retainer is also being used as a partial denture and carries a false tooth in an orthodontic-restorative case.

Disadvantages

- Do not have a very tight fit anteriorly. The fit and retention can be improved (see below,

acrylic facings), but is never as tight as with the VFRs.
- Costlier and more time-consuming to manufacture than VFRs.
- Poor at retaining any vertical tooth movements that may have been needed during more complex, fixed appliance orthodontic treatment.
- Poorer at maintaining space closure in spaced dentitions (e.g. hypodontia or diastema closure cases) than bonded retainers.

Components

The classic Hawley appliance comprises:

- Adams' clasps on UR6 and UL6 [0.7 mm stainless steel (ss)]
- Standard U-looped labial bow UR3 to UL3 (0.7 mm ss)
- Rests may also be incorporated to lie on the occlusal surfaces of the U7s (if erupted) to prevent their over-eruption. These are important if the appliance is to be worn full-time for any length of time
- Acrylic baseplate.

The identical design can be made for the lower arch.

However, modified designs are frequently used in present-day practice. These are aimed at overcoming some of the weaknesses inherent in the above design.

Variations
- **Use of acrylic facings on labial bows.** Frequently nowadays, clear, thin acrylic facing is incorporated onto both arches of the labial bow. Such facings straddle the labial bow wire by about 2 mm on either side. The facing runs between the mesial of each canine and transforms the bow into a close-fitting acrylic splint: the upper incisors and mesial of the canines are now sandwiched between the baseplate and the acrylic facing. As well as improving the fit, the facing also improves the anterior retention of the Hawley appliance.
- **'Wrap-around' modification.** This modification can be used in conjunction with an acrylic facing. Instead of the U-looped labial bow crossing the occlusal plane distal (usually) to the canines and mesial to the premolar, the bow, which is contoured to touch all the buccal surfaces of the teeth, extends and curls around the distal of the last standing molar at gingival level, i.e. no wire-work from the labial bow crosses the occlusal plane at a previous extraction site. This avoids the wire-work potentially wedging open any extraction spaces.

  The above design (known as a Begg wrap-around retainer) may, however, have relatively poor retention. Therefore, some operators may favour Adams' clasps on the U6s to which the 0.7-mm ss labial bow is soldered (via the clasp bridge). This design can again be combined with an acrylic facing. Once again, the whole arch is enclosed, anteriorly, posteriorly and laterally so that extraction spaces are encouraged to stay closed since no wire-work crosses the standard extraction sites.

Vacuum-formed retainers

Manufacture
- Special equipment is required as manufacture involves careful timing, heating and vacuum. Specifically, a vacuum-thermoforming machine is needed, which benefits from a two-stage motor that is said to help achieve maximum adaptation.
- In essence, a plastic sheet is placed over the appropriate working model for the retainer to be made. A number of different plastic grades exist that vary according to the thickness and properties required. For example, thicknesses vary from 0.5 to 3 mm with differing degrees of clarity or opacity. They vary in their durability from perhaps 1 to 2 years or so. Clearly, vacuum heat times will also be influenced by the thickness of the plastic, e.g. 20–50 seconds.
- The model needs to be cast from a hard material such as gypsum or high-quality stone. The sheet is heated up in a vacuum so that it is simultaneously softened and sucked down over the working model. Once the appropriate fit is achieved, the heat and vacuum automatically cut out and a freeze spray must be applied to rapidly cool the plastic. This prevents any more thinning from occurring once cooled and the effective shrinkage helps ensure a very close fit to the model. Once fully cooled, the (now) very tightly fitting sheet must be grossly trimmed initially and then carefully levered off the model.
- The retainer can then be finally trimmed so that the plastic extends just onto the gingival margins labially, lingually or palatally. Polishing or acrylic burs are used to smooth off the edges.
- In order to provide the laboratory prescription on a laboratory design card, this simply involves drawing an outline around the arch to indicate which teeth are to be included within the VFR. In many cases therefore, this drawn outline would include all the upper or lower teeth, including the second molars.

Advantages

- Much quicker and cheaper to make as they require far less hands-on technician time than, say, the manufacture of Hawley appliances.
- Should a re-make be required, then again this is easier and quicker to generate than a Hawley appliance.
- Easily the most aesthetic of the removable retainers and for this reason, appear to be very popular with patients.
- Can be used successfully for retaining overjet reduction as they act like a strap across the front of the upper incisors.
- A recent clinical trial (Rowland *et al.*, 2007) has shown VFRs to be slightly better at maintaining alignment of both upper and lower labial segments than Hawley retainers, at least over the initial 6-month period, and even though the Hawley retainers had acrylated labial bows. However, the difference was marginal in the upper labial segment.
- May be of help where patients have a significant gag reflex as they do not cover the palate.

Disadvantages

- Cover the occlusal surfaces of the teeth. Therefore, following active treatment, if further 'settling in' of the occlusion is required, then this is precluded during full-time wear of such appliances.
- Poor at retaining any vertical tooth movements that may have been needed during more complex, fixed appliance orthodontic treatment.
- Poorer at maintaining space closure in spaced dentitions (e.g. hypodontia or diastema closure cases) than bonded retainers.
- They should not be worn whilst eating as they will rapidly wear through. As with all retainers when not being worn, they should be kept in their own box for safe keeping (see below).

Variations

The main variant of this type of retainer is when a false tooth needs to be included, e.g. following avulsion of a tooth or in hypodontia cases (see Figure 7.3b–d). This modification can be very aesthetic, but if patients eat with a VFR in place, they are likely to wear the retainer out very quickly. Indeed, all VFRs should *always be taken out for eating and drinking* due to the risk of sugary/acidic liquids otherwise bathing the teeth for long periods of time, leading to a very high caries and erosion risk. However, whilst retainers are not being worn, teeth can and likely will move (often much more quickly than when active tooth movement was being undertaken with appliances). This can then defeat the object of treatment if space is lost.

Bonded (or fixed) retainers

Most bonded retainers are made of multi-strand (or co-axial) stainless steel (ss) wires. These consist of multiple, very thin, ss wires that are intertwined to form a single, thin archwire. The diameters of the individual wires vary, as does the overall thickness of the wire. However, generally a round cross-sectional, multi-strand wire is used whose overall thickness is between 0.0175 and 0.022 inches. Figure 7.4 shows an example of an upper bonded retainer.

Bonded retainers are usually cemented canine-to-canine on each tooth (either on the lower or upper arch, or both arches). Therefore, these multi-strand wires offer a small amount of flexibility (allowing physiological movement) between each tooth. This makes debonds less likely – in contrast to previous retainers which used a solid length of small diameter wire.

The laboratory card prescription is often very simple: a line is drawn across the lingual or palatal surfaces of the teeth to be included in the bonded retainer. If there are any specific points that need to be made with regard to positioning, these can be stated in the prescription notes. For example, 'Please make a 0.0175″ bonded retainer from UR3 to UL3. Please site it incisally especially on UR12 and UL12 to keep it clear of the occlusion'.

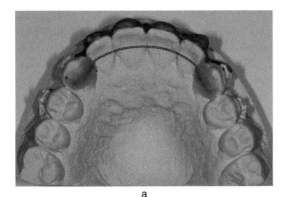

a

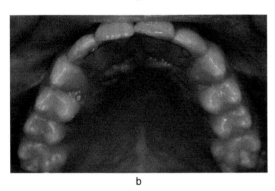

b

Figure 7.4 Example of an upper bonded retainer, waxed onto the working model, ready for placement clinically (a). An upper bonded retainer in place intraorally (b).

Using light curing technology, such retainers are bonded to the lingual or palatal surface of the teeth it is desired to 'retain' – in practice, often (though not always) from the upper canine-to-canine or lower canine-to-canine (i.e. 3–3). The composite used is the same as that used for the bonding of brackets. A careful technique is required as it is essential that the retainer should be held securely in place during bonding (to avoid any risk of inhalation or swallowing). In addition, a completely dry field is required for secure bonding and it is vital to ensure the bonding composite is maintained on the appropriate palatal or lingual surface, i.e. it should not be allowed to penetrate between the teeth;

occlusally or onto the gingivae. Any such 'escape' must be thoroughly cleaned away so that the patient's teeth or periodontal condition are not compromised, and so that flossing can still be undertaken using a floss threader. See Chapter 8 for details on the fitting of bonded retainers.

Removable versus fixed retainers

Many patients (and indeed many dentists and even orthodontists) will consider that a bonded retainer is certain to be a better retainer than a removable retainer. The truth, however, is somewhat different and the evidence is not yet available to recommend one over the other.

Furthermore, in some instances a removable retainer must be used, whilst in others a bonded retainer has to be used. For example, a bonded retainer cannot hold overjet reduction satisfactorily, since the lower lip can still trap behind the upper incisors and move them all forward – regardless of the fact that teeth are bonded together. Similarly, removable retainers cannot hold significant spacing closed. This is because it is not realistic to expect patients to wear removable retainers indefinitely on a full-time basis. Indeed, long-term full-time wear would not even be desirable, since dental and periodontal health would likely be compromised. In any case, and particularly in the case of Hawley appliances, appearance would always be compromised, which would defeat the major aim of most orthodontic treatment. Hence, when removable retainers are used, there is far more opportunity for spacing to relapse during the periods when the appliance is not being worn. Of course, the same can be true of a bonded retainer if it debonds; but in theory at least, whilst bonded, it should hold spacing closed.

However, whilst evidence is lacking with regard to which is the 'best retainer', it is still possible to consider the advantages and disadvantages of the three main retainer types. Table 7.1 highlights some major differences between

Table 7.1 A brief personal overview of retainer types in 'consumer report' style.

Type of retainer	Maintenance of alignment	Maintenance of overjet reduction	Ease of adjustment/ repair or remake	Fail safe – for dental health (i.e. patient can remove appliance)	Allows settling	Ability to hold spaces closed or hold periodontally involved cases	Wear and tear resistance	Aesthetic quality
Hawley	√	√√	√√	√√	√√√	XXX	√√	XXX
Essix	√√	√√	√√	√√	√	XXX	√√	√√
Bonded	√√√	XXX	XXX	XXX	X	√√ (theoretically for spaces)	√ (failure rates of 15–40% reported)	√√

the retainer types and, combined with the earlier discussion regarding maturational change, hopefully clarifies why it is not possible to guarantee perfectly aligned/positioned teeth forever to everyone.

Retention regimes

Having dealt with why we need retainers, the types of retainers and their strengths and weaknesses, the next thing to consider is how often and for how long the patient should wear them. We also consider other points such as how to care for retainers.

Retention regimes can be classified in a number of different ways. The classification suggested here is based on type of tooth movement related to length of wear. Furthermore, it is probably fair to say that the length of time of wear (in terms of months or years) is increasingly influenced by patients' wishes.

For example, many patients, when they learn that teeth tend to move throughout life, tending to crowd with age (regardless of whether orthodontic treatment has been undertaken or not), now ask whether they can continue wearing their retainers on a long-term basis. This may certainly be feasible in many cases, but probably not all. The reason is that long-term or indefinite wear of a retainer can, just as an active brace can, damage the teeth/periodontal condition if good oral hygiene, sensible diet and regular attendance is not maintained. Therefore, for some patients, it may be in their best interests to advise against indefinite retainer wear. This important subject will be discussed further in the contra-indications section below.

Retention following simple, limited tooth movement

This may involve a patient wearing a custom-made, removable retainer or passive removable appliance for only a short time, and would apply to uncomplicated cases involving limited tooth movements and where other tooth positions are accepted.

Pushing teeth over the bite

In a few interceptive cases where an incisor(s) has been pushed over the bite using a URA, the overbite may be tenuous once a positive overjet has been achieved. In these cases, there is initially unlikely to be sufficient overbite for 'natural retention' (see below). In this situation, it would be sensible to remove all posterior capping (to encourage teeth to come into occlusion), but to ask the patient to continue wearing the URA full-time until their next review appointment. At this point therefore, providing the tooth/teeth have been moved sufficiently forward, the spring or screw should be left passive for this visit, so that the appliance is functioning solely as a retainer.

At the next review, the occlusion should be re-assessed and the overbite measured once more. If this is still tenuous, then it may be appropriate to ask the patient to wear the appliance at night only for one or two more follow-up visits. This would mean the anterior tooth/teeth is/are 'reminded' or encouraged to remain anteriorly positioned, but the teeth are given maximal opportunity to erupt toward one another so that the overbite can be more fully re-established.

If at further follow-up the overbite is found still not to be sufficient to maintain crossbite correction, then the appliance will have to be withdrawn, accepting the likelihood of some, if not total, relapse. However, this begs the question as to whether the treatment should have been attempted/was appropriate in the first place. This may also be affected by the information given to patients/parents/guardians regarding the likely outcome of treatment during the consenting process. What is not acceptable is for a young child to be forced or asked to wear an appliance indefinitely as a retainer to make up for the inadequacies of the operator's diagnostic abilities.

Where a posterior crossbite has been corrected with a URA, it would normally be appropriate to ask the patient to continue wearing the appliance full-time at least up until the first visit following correction of the crossbite. However, at that stage, the posterior capping should be removed to encourage the buccal teeth to come into occlusion. Any springs or screws should be left passive at this time too. The positions of the buccal teeth should be reassessed at future visits, but once the teeth are inter-digitated, then the appliance can be discarded. For cases involving removable appliances, a retention period of more than 6 months seems excessive, since such cases should normally only involve crossbites requiring 2–3 mm of buccal tooth movement, i.e. relatively small amounts of tipping.

Simple, single-arch fixed appliance cases

Cases that involve a single-arch fixed appliance, where, for example, only buccally crowded canines have been aligned, may be entirely suitable for such simple retention as only the aligned canines need any retention (if little or no movement of other teeth has been necessary). In such cases, removable retainer wear would seem entirely suitable and the regime might be full-time wear for several nights and then nights only for 6 months. The appliance could probably then be discarded if wished.

Retention following fixed appliances (multiple tooth movements)

Following upper and lower fixed appliance treatment, patients are usually advised to wear a retainer for a year or more, since most, if not all, teeth will have been subjected to orthodontic forces and moved from their original positions. The retainers used may be either removable (e.g. vacuum-formed) or bonded. Currently, there is no regime of wear that has been deemed to be clearly superior to any other. So, for example, some clinicians may advise a patient to wear a removable retainer full-time for 6 months and then suggest nights-only wear for another 6 months to a year. Others may advise nights-only wear from the outset and for at least a year. Of course, there are other variations along these lines. However, recently, the first randomised clinical study to assess two different regimes found that nights-only wear of removable retainers from the outset of retention provided as much stability as full-time wear after 6 months. It is possible therefore, that in future, nights-only wear may become the regime of choice, at least in routine orthodontic cases, i.e. treatments not involving inter-disciplinary treatment or where special risks apply.

What is more generally agreed is that:

- A minimum of 1 year's retention is recommended, providing oral hygiene/dental health allow this.
- The period of nights-only wear is extensive.
- Pre-treatment spacing, posterior crossbite correction and/or rotations generally mean that the retention period overall is likely to be longer as these tooth positions are known to be particularly prone to relapse.
- Use of removable retainers allows wear to be reduced or maintained according to how the teeth settle. For example, if all is going well after 8 or 9 months of nights-only wear, alternate-nights wear might be advised.

Liaison with the specialist: why do we need to know what is being retained?

It is unlikely that any orthodontist can follow-up every patient they have treated on a very long-term basis. Indeed, it is generally accepted that patients will have to be discharged back to their own dentist post-orthodontic treatment. However, a problem is increasingly arising since more and more patients (anecdotally at least) seem to want to carry on wearing their retainers beyond the initial year after appliance removal. Therefore, it is common practice for the orthodontist to discharge the patient back to their own dentist, *assuming that the dentist will be willing and able to take over the care and responsibility for monitoring their patient's retainer(s).* However, assumptions can be dangerous so the following procedure would be seen as the ideal and is recommended when feasible and where all the following apply:

- It is confirmed that a patient wishes to continue wearing retainers
- The patient has demonstrated that they are able to maintain good dental health
- The patient has experienced few or no breakages or appliance losses
- The patient has attended checks regularly.

The orthodontist should discharge the patient with a covering letter to the dentist. This letter should include:

- A summary of the initial malocclusion and brief treatment.
- When active treatment was completed.
- The type(s) of retainer(s) fitted and the instructions on wear and care the patient has been given, e.g. the patient has been fitted with upper and lower VFRs which they have been advised to wear on alternate nights for as long as they would like to keep their teeth as straight as possible.
- Advise regarding the frequency of retainer check, e.g. every 6 months.
- It is also good practice if the orthodontist highlights particular points to check, e.g.
  - Assess the retainer fit
  - Assess for breakages – these may be subtle, particularly bonded retainer debonds. In such cases a composite 'blob' commonly debonds from a tooth, leaving an air gap

of less than 0.5 mm, which may be evident to the naked eye only when air is blown around the composite and a tell-tale margin of moisture is seen glistening between the palatal/lingual enamel and the composite blob.
  - Assess the dental and gingival health; if there is bleeding on probing or any caries, is this caused by or exacerbated by the retainer wear? Can the problem be rectified, e.g. dietary or oral hygiene measures; providing hygienist appointments?
  - Other information, such as tips on repairing bonded retainers, can also be helpful.
- The orthodontist should indicate to the dentist under what circumstances the retainers should be stopped and discarded (in the case of removable retainers) or removed (in the case of fixed retainers). For example, where a dental health problem associated with the retainer(s) cannot be resolved, then it is best to advise the patient's dentist to stop retention and discard or remove the appliances in the best interests of the patient's dental health. This would mean that the possibility of increased tooth movement would have to be accepted, but this would be preferable to compromising dental health and potentially jeopardising the longevity of a tooth or teeth. Likewise, should a patient request the retainer(s) to be stopped or removed, then the patient would have to accept the possibility of more tooth movement occurring. In either case, it is not usually sensible to offer re-treatment or further orthodontic treatment should further tooth movement occur post-retention.

In general, when patients are discharged back to their dentist, they are likely to be wearing removable retainers at least 2 or 3 nights per week and/or a bonded retainer in one or both arches.

An ideal retention regime with removable retainers has yet to be defined based on scientific evidence. However, after about a year's retention, if the patient wishes and is able to continue on a long-term basis with removable retainer wear, then, based on personal experience, it seems that wear 2–3 nights per week is a reasonable regime; retainer wear, say, only 1 night per week, seems to increase the likelihood of tooth movement. Also, most patients who want to carry on wearing retainers seem to find a regular habit helpful in maintaining wear and find 2 or 3 nights per week acceptable. For others, continuing wear each and every night might be preferable if it maintains the habit more reliably.

Contra-indications to retention

Since URA treatment is almost entirely aimed at interceptive treatment, nowadays only a few situations remain where some form of retention will be needed. However, should the patient fall into one of the categories described below, or a similar one, then, as with fixed appliances, retention would be contra-indicated.

Ideally, every patient who has undergone fixed appliance orthodontic treatment would benefit from retention for a minimum of about 1 year. However, there are some exceptions where a period of retention is likely to be impractical or frankly contra-indicated:

- Patients where treatment has had to be abandoned early due to poor oral hygiene.
- Patients who have sustained such frequent breakages during active treatment that treatment has had to be abandoned early.

In these circumstances, since treatment has not been completed, it is also likely that the tooth positions will be very unstable. There is therefore little or no point in trying to 'settle' the teeth, since their stability will not increase. Furthermore, where, for example, the occlusion may benefit from greater inter-digitation, i.e. upper and lower buccal teeth may benefit from being free from any occlusal coverage, in order to allow them to move toward each other, then

a retainer may actually prevent such potentially helpful, spontaneous change. Similarly, there may be situations where a small amount of space reduction occurs naturally, but this will be impeded by a retainer.

Other cases where retention may be contra-indicated include:

- Patients in whom significant demineralisation/caries has been found at debond beneath/around the appliances.
- Patient attendance has been so poor that supervision of retainer appliance wear is likely to be severely compromised, bringing with it the risk of damage to dental health if wear will probably be mostly or entirely unsupervised.

In some patients of course, retainers may be fitted as usual at the end of active treatment, but later withdrawn in exactly the same way as active treatment may be terminated early. Usually this occurs when dental health problems arise during the retention period and the patient is unable (or unwilling) to address these even with support.

'Natural' retention

This refers to the one instance where retention may not be required. Yes, it can happen! The one time it can be said with certainty that retention is redundant is when an incisor(s) has been pushed over the bite and there is sufficient overbite to hold the correction (at least 2 mm of overbite is present). At this point the URA has done its job and further wear is pointless, since it is the overbite that will hold the correction or not.

Reference

Rowland H, Hichens L, Williams A, *et al.* (2007) The effectiveness of Hawley and vacuum-formed retainers: a single-center randomized controlled trial. *American Journal of Orthodontics and Dentofacial Orthopedics* **132** (6), 730–737.

Fitting and Checking Retainers

8

This chapter will provide guidance on what should be checked once retainers have been fitted following the end of active treatment. It will be assumed that treatment has been completed satisfactorily as planned and that two-arch fixed appliances have been used.

Many operators will not see the patient again for about 3 months after retainers are fitted. Ideally, it might be argued that an earlier check (perhaps 4–6 weeks after the retainers have first been fitted) would ensure that there are no problems or misunderstandings with retainer wear at this crucial stage of treatment. Unfortunately, should either the patient or operator not appreciate this, then an entire 2-year treatment can easily be rendered useless due to poor or no retainer wear leading to rapid and gross relapse. It is therefore extremely important that operators ensure that patients are aware of the need and importance of the retention period.

Learning outcomes

At the end of this chapter you should:

- Be able to explain the importance of regular retainer checks to patients
- Have the knowledge to be able to undertake a retainer check
- Have the knowledge to undertake simple retainer adjustments

First fitting of removable retainers

When the appliance is received from the laboratory, as with any appliance, basic checks should be undertaken to confirm:

- It is the correct appliance for the patient
- It is the prescription requested
- The appliance fits the model correctly

Orthodontic Retainers and Removable Appliances: Principles of Design and Use, First Edition.
Friedy Luther and Zararna Nelson-Moon.
© 2013 Friedy Luther and Zararna Nelson-Moon. Published 2013 by Blackwell Publishing Ltd.

- There are no obvious deformities in the working model. This is not always possible to assess for VFRs, since the model may have been destroyed when the appliance was removed from it.

In addition, once the above are confirmed as correct, the appliance should be checked to see there are no sharp edges or acrylic 'blips', which may cause discomfort or damage to the patient (see Chapter 4).

Checking the fit of Hawley retainers in the mouth (see Chapter 4)

The appliance should seat down fully around the teeth and the labial bow (modified with or without an acrylic facing) should fit snugly against the teeth without any obvious air gaps between the wire and the teeth or between the acrylic facing (if used) and teeth.

Appliance not seating down fully

If well made, these appliances should fit down properly. However, occasionally the appliance may not seat down fully if the colleting has not been sufficiently trimmed from around the teeth. If this occurs, often further trimming is needed in the premolar or molar region. You will need to check how far occlusally the acrylic lies. If it is preventing full seating, then an acrylic bur and straight handpiece should be used to trim the acrylic in the colleted areas such that the collets rise only to about half way along the palatal surfaces of, for example, the premolars and/or first permanent molars.

Another reason the appliance may not seat fully is if acrylic has crept along the arms of the fly-overs between the contact points. In this circumstance, Adams' pliers can be used to simply 'crunch' off any stray acrylic by squeezing the acrylic between the beaks of the pliers.

Where any acrylic is to be trimmed, this should of course be done outside the mouth. The patient, nurse and operator should wear eye protection whilst trimming is being undertaken.

Appliance loose

If the appliance fits properly, but is loose, there are usually two simple solutions:

- Consider tightening the Adams' clasps to engage the undercuts more deeply using Adams' pliers. This should be done by gripping each of the fly-overs in turn at the most buccal point and bending the arrowheads downward so that they engage the undercuts more.
- Either alternatively or in addition to the Adams' clasp adjustment, it may be necessary to adjust the labial bow. This will depend on where the appliance is loose.

Figure 8.1 demonstrates a poorly fitting, loose labial bow and how to adjust it. As shown, once the retention has been improved, the final adjustment that may be required is to reposition the labial bow. This is sometimes needed due to the fact that when the U-loops are tightened, this tends to move the labial bow incisally. This can only be tolerated for a small number of visits since the bow will gradually edge toward the incisor tips. This will lead to poor retention and, with a Hawley retainer in the lower arch, potentially occlusal interferences with the upper teeth. In order to avoid this, a simple adjustment needs to be made in the U-loop such that the anterior part of the bow is pushed gingivally. This is done using Adams' pliers to push the mesial component of the wire (which projects anterior to the U-loop) in a gingival direction so that the labial bow lies in the middle of the incisor crowns or as close to this as possible.

Appliance not fitting

If a new appliance simply does not fit, despite undertaking the checking and adjustments

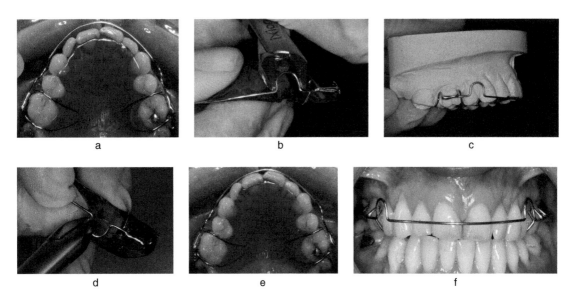

Figure 8.1 A poorly fitting, loose labial bow (a). To tighten the labial bow, the U-loops of the labial bow are gently squeezed using either Adams' pliers or spring-forming pliers: place the U-loop between the beaks and squeeze gently so the U-loop closes or tightens a little (b). This should bring the labial bow into closer contact with the teeth; this should be done carefully and relatively symmetrically, so that the bow does not distort to one side – leading to no fit at all. Once the retention has been improved, the final adjustment that may be required is to reposition the labial bow. This is sometimes needed due to the fact that when the U-loops are tightened, this tends to move the labial bow incisally (c and d). This should bring the labial bow into closer contact with the teeth, but again this should be done carefully and relatively symmetrically, so that the bow does not distort to one side – leading to no fit at all. The improved fit is shown (e and f). (Photographs courtesy of Simon Littlewood and Carol Bentley.)

described above, the fit on the working model should be checked. If it fits the model well, but not the mouth, then it may be that:

- A tooth or teeth have moved since the impression was taken, or
- The impression was dragged or has otherwise been distorted, either at the time it was taken or at some point subsequently.

Any such scenario will mean a re-make with a new impression is needed.

Checking the fit of vacuum-formed retainers

The appliance should seat down fully around the teeth and there should be no rebound as it is seated. The margin of the appliance extends just onto the gingivae, buccally and palatally/lingually, in both arches. These appliances will normally fit very tightly, so to avoid surprising the patient, they should be advised of this before you actually fit them.

As you push the appliance down over the teeth, be vigilant: if on fitting down, the appliance is seen to be forcibly pressing against the gingivae (causing blanching), stop and remove the appliance as this is likely to be painful for the patient; it will need easing in those areas before attempting the fit again. The appliance can be trimmed with scissors and then smoothed with a greenstone in a straight handpiece if it is extended excessively onto the gingivae and engages undercuts. Alternatively, or as well, it may need easing on the inner (fit) surface, again using a greenstone. Care should be taken when easing the appliance as the material is thin and it is easy to pierce it.

Once the appliance is seated, ask the patient whether there are any particular areas that feel much tighter than elsewhere or whether any points actually feel sore. If so, the above adjustments may be needed once more. In addition, with the appliance in place, look around the appliance and check whether the gingivae are blanching. If there are any such areas, again easing as above will be needed. Figure 8.2 shows actual trauma caused by a new vacuum-formed retainer (VFR) being fitted following debond. If during the fitting of the appliance it becomes clear that the appliance simply will not fit down or fails to seat down fully, despite

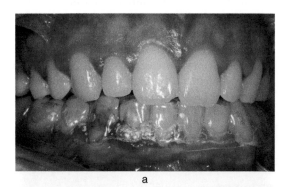

a

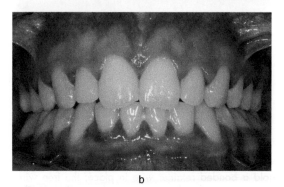

b

Figure 8.2 This vacuum-formed retainer (VFR), just fitted at debond, is causing not just blanching of the gingivae but actual bleeding (a). However, it is very clear where easing is needed once the VFR is removed (b).

the adjustments noted previously, then, as with a Hawley retainer, it suggests either:

* A tooth or teeth have moved since the impression was taken, or
* The impression was dragged or has otherwise been distorted, either at the time it was taken or at some point subsequently.

Any such scenario will mean a re-make and a new impression will be needed.

Checking and fitting bonded retainers

Checking bonded retainers

Bonded retainers should be checked in the mouth before they are cemented.

It is essential to check that they:

* Fit closely to the lingual or palatal surfaces of the relevant teeth
* Are as far away from the gingivae as possible (but not visible when viewed from the front) to maximise the patient's ability to clean effectively
* Are not active appliances
* Are not interfering with the occlusion.

Should any problems be evident with regard to any of the above factors, then either adjustment or a re-make is required.

Before any bonded retainer is placed, the occlusion should be checked – to see that there is room for the retainer; this is obviously necessary for upper bonded retainers. This should be done before active treatment is completed and before the fixed appliances are removed. If necessary, the overbite may need to be reduced further to allow a bonded retainer to be fitted.

Before a bonded retainer is to be bonded into position, it should first be checked carefully for fit in the mouth. It is essential thoroughly to dry the relevant teeth beforehand and the retainer can then be carefully placed into position whilst holding it tightly in mosquito forceps or fingertips. The wire should sit appropriately against the teeth with a minimal air gap. Should it not sit properly, then a decision has to be made whether the wire can be adjusted at the chairside or whether a new retainer needs to be made.

Fitting (bonding) bonded retainers

Various techniques can be used to help locate the retainer securely whilst bonding:

- **Use of floss.** Lengths of floss are placed inter-proximally through at least two of the contacts across which the retainer wire is to run; the retainer is then carefully held in place whilst one floss length at a time is looped back through the contact so that the retainer wire has floss running under and over it. The floss should be placed so that it loops over the retainer wire and can be pulled tight on the labial side of the anterior teeth. Once several such loops are in place, they are pulled tight (all from the labial side), thus trapping the wire, hopefully in the correct place.
- **Intra-oral orthodontic elastics.** These are used in a similar way to dental floss, and are placed between at least two pairs of the teeth to be bonded. The teeth selected should be at opposite ends of those to be bonded, and the small elastics are stretched over each selected tooth crown so that they lie just below the contact point before the retainer is positioned. The retainer is then carefully positioned by hand whilst each elastic is then pulled back over the crown from the palatal or lingual to the buccal aspect, trapping the wire on the palatal or lingual surface. Intermediate teeth may also need to be engaged, depending on how well the retainer 'locks' into place once the elastics are looped back over the crowns, trapping the wire in the appropriate position. Bonding can then safely proceed, using the acid-etch technique.
- **Use of custom-made jigs.** In this option, the retainer sits in a jig whilst it is bonded to

several of the teeth. The jig is custom-made and designed to sit largely on the lingual or palatal aspects of the teeth. However, a lip extends onto the labial aspect so as to seat the jig definitively into the correct place. These jigs can be easy to use and hold the retainer in place safely and securely whilst it is being bonded using the acid-etch technique.

Assuming the wire retainer is to be bonded to the lingual surface of each tooth (from canine to canine), then the jig is usually constructed to engage and cover the wire on the lingual/palatal aspect of the central incisors. Therefore, each end of the retainer is exposed and it is straightforward to bond these free ends to the canine teeth (with or without the lateral incisors), whilst the retainer is held securely in position by the jig. The jig is only removed once the retainer has been bonded to the teeth that are not covered by it. Care must be taken to ensure the jig is carefully constructed so that it peels away easily at that stage – without of course debonding the teeth which have already had the bonded retainer bonded to them. An example of a silicone putty jig is shown in Figure 8.3.

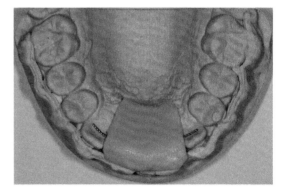

Figure 8.3 A silicone putty jig can be used to safely hold a bonded retainer wire in place; the free wire ends are bonded first to secure the retainer to the teeth. The jig is designed so that it may then be peeled away, revealing the remainder of the wire. This can then be bonded to the lingual/palatal surfaces without the risk of the retainer falling off.

Various jig designs exist, e.g. acrylic jigs or those made from a silicone impression material. The latter are becoming increasingly popular as they are cheap, easy to make and mould well to the teeth. Their inherent flexibility also allows somewhat easier 'peeling' of the jig from the wire than a rigid, acrylic jig might.

More precise details of such techniques can be found in the references at the end of this chapter.

Once the bonded retainer has been bonded into place, it is essential to check the interproximal contacts using floss. Specially strengthened or stiffened lengths of floss can be threaded gingivally to the wire to clean this area, but also to check the contact at this level is clear of composite. Ordinary floss can be used to check the contact incisal to the wire. Should any composite be detected, it is essential to remove it to avoid it acting as a plaque trap. Composite-removing burs in a right-angled handpiece can be used to do this, as well as scalers.

As noted previously, as well as checking the occlusion before any bonded retainer is fitted to ensure there is room for it, a further essential check must occur once the bonded retainer has been placed. This is to check that the retainer is not interfering with the occlusion. To assess this, the patient should be asked to close their teeth together and chew around onto some articulating paper. Any high spots that show up should be removed. The paper should be re-inserted until such time as no high spots are visible or are extremely faint, and the patient confirms their bite feels satisfactory and there are no sharp surfaces (Figure 8.4).

Follow-up visits: is the retention working?

Once retainers of any sort have been fitted, it is essential to arrange appropriate follow-up. It is not good practice or ethical either to simply send the patient away with instructions in the hope that they will follow these without ques-

tion, or to simply discharge the patient back to their own dentist in the hope they will monitor the patient's retainers (see Chapter 7 with regard to managing the transfer of care back to the patient's own dentist).

Whoever has undertaken the active orthodontic treatment should follow up the patient, ideally for a year. We will first discuss the follow-up 'regime' and then discuss what should be checked at follow-up to confirm the retention is 'working'.

Follow-up visits

The suggested follow-up 'regime' is:

1. Once the retainers have been fitted and instructions for wear and care provided, the patient should be seen again a few weeks later and certainly after 3 months. Retention is an essential and critical part of treatment and this should be re-iterated and emphasised to the patient. As already highlighted, if the patient fails to wear their retainers as (hopefully) appropriately instructed, they can be back at square one in a very short period of time. By seeing the patient within a few weeks of the retainers being fitted, the operator will have a chance to deal with any problems or misunderstandings on the part of the patient before anything too detrimental occurs. It perhaps also sends a re-inforcing message to the patient that this stage is really important and that matters can easily slip if instructions are not followed.

   Putting off this initial review beyond 3 months is excessive. Initial reviews beyond this time really leave no slack to allow correction of any misunderstandings about wear and mean any inadvertent trauma caused by any form of removable retainer cannot be intercepted. These issues may mean the appliance is not being worn adequately and by the time the patient returns, any relapse may be well underway.

2. If all is progressing satisfactorily at visit 1, then it is reasonable to lengthen appoint-

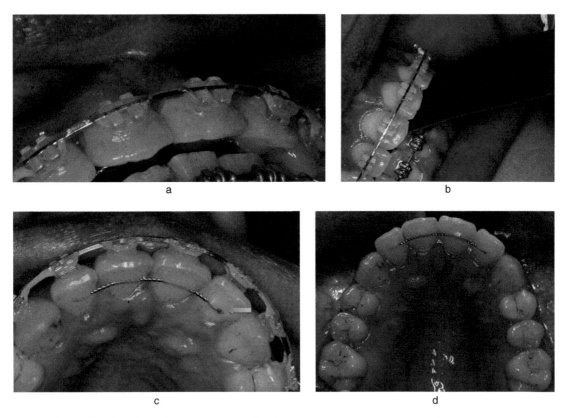

Figure 8.4 Checking the occlusion on a newly bonded retainer. A lower incisor can be seen to be in contact with one of the composite blobs (a). To demonstrate such 'high spots' more clearly, articulating paper is used and the patient asked to 'chew around' (b). The high spot is identified (arrowed, c) and then relieved using a composite removing burr (d). Of course, more than one high spot may exist and these must all be relieved. In this case the fixed appliance has then been debonded. (Photographs courtesy of Simon Littlewood.)

ment intervals to about 3 or sometimes 6 months. However, it is good practice to advise the patient that should there be any problems between visits, then they should contact you as soon as possible so that any issues can be dealt with. It is much better to see the patient sooner rather than later in these circumstances since, for example, should an appliance become loose or break, then the teeth may well start to move. The situation may become irretrievable if the patient fails to return for weeks or months. In contrast, an early return may allow adjustment(s) to be done before anything much has happened.

3. If all is well at visit 2, then it is suggested that 3- or even 6-monthly follow-up is main-

tained. However, the caveat should always remain: that should there be any problems at all between visits, then the patient should contact you as soon as possible so that any issues can be dealt with.

What to check

At the first follow-up, it is advisable to ask the patient:

- How they are getting on with the retainers
- Whether they are having any problems with the retainers
- How much they are wearing them (beware: do not ask leading questions such as 'Are

you wearing the retainers every night like I said,' as this will beg the answer 'Yes' even when it may not be true).

If the patient reports no problems, the next step is:

- To check yourself that the retainers fit well, and
- In the case of removable retainers, check they are not causing irritation/ulceration, e.g. around the lingual frenum. The patient may be unaware of any rubbing here or elsewhere. Should there be any sign of ulceration, then the retainer should be eased.

Oral hygiene

Next, no matter what sort of retainer is being checked, another vital step is to assess the patient's oral hygiene. A periodontal probe should be used to check for areas of bleeding on probing; any plaque build up should be noted plus a visual assessment of gingival condition should be undertaken, e.g. any swelling or redness should be noted. It is then necessary to inform the patient of your findings and, if needed, arrange scaling and oral hygiene instruction. Good oral hygiene should always be commented on and encouraged. However, should oral hygiene be poor, or relatively so (keeping in mind that any orthodontic appliance automatically renders the oral cavity high risk for dental disease), then steps should not only be taken to address this but also to monitor and document the situation. For example, if following any appropriate hygienist visit, oral hygiene remains poor, this cannot be ignored. Indeed, it may become necessary to consider treatment termination. Suggestions for how this could be managed and the steps leading up to this are outlined in Chapter 9.

Retention of the retainer

The retention of the appliances should be checked next. There is little that can be done to improve retention in the case of VFRs, emphasising how important it is to check that the fit of the appliance is optimal when it is first fitted. If it was, but fit is being lost after even just one visit, it suggests that the patient may not be wearing the appliance as instructed. This is a reasonable assumption since, as has already been said, the teeth are at their most unstable as active treatment is completed and the active appliances are removed. Bone and gingivae will have had no opportunity to consolidate and therefore the teeth will easily and rapidly relapse without appropriate retainer wear. Clearly, this would need to be discussed with the patient/parent/guardian to find out what has prevented the retainers from being worn. If the patient has simply chosen not to wear them, then the consequences need to be spelled out once again, making it clear that the patient needs to take responsibility for their own decision, since re-treatment would not normally be countenanced.

In the case of Hawley retainers (unlike VFRs), retention often reduces between appointments, since as with any other removable appliance, insertion and removal result in slight flexing of the clasps and other components and thus gradual loss of retention. Retention can however normally be improved, simply by adjusting the Adams' clasps and labial bow as described previously.

Care of the retainer

For bonded retainers, of course, patient cooperation centres around the care of the retainers rather than the wear. Very careful examination needs to take place to check no debonds have occurred (Figure 8.5). Initially, simple visual inspection may show up any gross deformation of the wire or debonds where the tooth has moved a millimetre or more from the wire. However, more frequently when a debond occurs, the air gap between the tooth surface and failed composite may be minute. This can generally only be seen by blowing air around each of the composite blobs and seeing if a

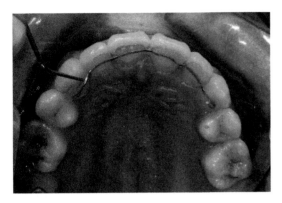

Figure 8.5 Example of a debonded composite 'blob' on an upper bonded retainer. The air gap between the tooth surface and failed composite may be minute, and is often only detected by blowing air around each composite blob and seeing if a salivary film is visible between the tooth surface and fit surface of the failed composite. In this case, a sharp probe has helped detect the failure by running it around the edge of each composite blob. *Note*: the patient is frequently completely unaware of such a debond. The bonded retainer shown here is an older form made of a single, solid (rather than multi-stranded) wire.

salivary film is visible between the tooth surface and fit surface of the failed composite. In addition, a sharp probe should be used as an extra aid as this may also help detect a gap by running it around the edge of each composite blob. Occasionally, composite staining can be a clue to suggest that a debond has occurred but this takes time to develop.

Should a debond be found, its repair is described in Chapter 9.

What to measure

Ultimately, of course, we need to assess whether the retainer is doing its job. This means we need to measure and assess whether the occlusion and alignment are being maintained as planned. This can only properly be done if it is known what the original malocclusion was as what is being retained needs to be known.

For example, if the patient had a Class I malocclusion prior to orthodontic correction, the main factor being retained and which should be checked during retention is the good tooth alignment, since it is unlikely that the patient will develop an overjet. On the other hand, if the patient had a Class II division 1 malocclusion prior to correction, then assessing the stability of overjet reduction is clearly essential.

Other more subtle aspects may need to be assessed. For example, in patients where palatally ectopic canines have been aligned, then as well as general alignment assessment, it is also important to assess the overbite associated with the previously ectopic canine. The tooth will normally have been placed in a Class I occlusion relative to the lower canine. However, contraction of the scar tissue in the palate (from the surgery to expose the canine) can cause some relapse in the canine position; specifically it can result in the canine being intruded so that the overbite reduces. If the patient is wearing a removable retainer, this will not prevent this reduction in overbite from occurring since removable retainers alone cannot retain teeth that are moving in the vertical dimension. The risk therefore is that the tooth may relapse into crossbite, since the reducing overbite will be insufficient to counteract any 'palatal pull' from any contracting scar tissue. In this situation then, the overbite needs to be assessed from visit to visit and if the clinician is unaware of what the presenting malocclusion was, then this would be missed. Furthermore, the reduction in overbite over time would almost certainly not be noticed until too late. Early recognition however, would allow a bonded retainer to be placed before the lack of overbite allows a crossbite to occur, assuming dental health allows.

Overall then, it is recommended that clinicians:

- Be aware or find out what the presenting malocclusion was
- Assess and note the alignment of the teeth at each follow-up visit

- Note any changes in overjet
- Note whether any extraction spaces (if relevant) are opening up
- Note any changes in the occlusion, e.g. changes in buccal segment relationships.

Other points to note will depend on what the presenting malocclusion was.

Long-term follow-up

Removable retainers

After about a year, if the patient wishes to continue retainer wear or if it would be advisable for them to do so (always with the caveat that dental health is maintained and co-operation allows it), then the amount of retainer wear can often be reduced. Alternate-night long-term wear may be quite satisfactory rather than continuing with every–night wear. Wearing retainers on only 1 night per week seems inadequate to minimise tooth movement in most cases. Twice-yearly retainer checks would generally seem reasonable, but for some patients an annual retainer check may be perfectly satisfactory, providing the patient is aware they can make contact sooner should any problems develop.

Bonded retainers

After the first year of satisfactory wear (meaning no or possibly only one breakage and maintenance of good dental health), review could probably be annual. Again, this assumes that the patient is aware they can make contact sooner should any problems develop.

Alternatively, where a patient has had more frequent problems, then depending on the type and extent of these, follow-up may need to be more frequent, but this cannot usually be sustained for long periods. Therefore, should problems persist, a decision needs to be taken as to whether the retention should be terminated.

The problems associated with retainers and retainer wear are discussed in more detail in Chapter 9.

References

Hobson RS, Eastaugh DP (1993) A silicone putty splint for rapid placement of directly bonded retainers. *Journal of Clinical Orthodontics* **27**, 536–537.

Shah AA, Sandler PJ, Murray AM (2005) How to . . . place a lower bonded retainer. *Journal of Orthodontics* **32**, 206–210.

Fitting a fixed/bonded retainer. Available at http://www.ncl.ac.uk/dental/ortho/Ret-fix.htm (accessed 13 August 2012).

Problems with Retainers and Trouble-shooting

The previous chapters on retainers and retention have discussed why retainers are needed; the different types of retainer; how they are checked and fitted; and what needs to be checked at follow-up. We now discuss what can happen during the the long-term follow-up of retainers; what can go wrong and what – if anything – can be done to deal with these problems.

Learning outcomes

By the end of this chapter you should be able to:

- Explain the main problems associated with retention and retainers
- Advise patients how to manage problems with retainers
- Explain to patients what, realistically, they may expect from orthodontic treatment during and following retention
- Explain to patients why retention may need to be terminated

Problems with removable retainers and trouble-shooting

The problems that can arise with removable retainers can be grouped in a variety of ways. However, a convenient, but also clinically realistic, way of classifying the problems is as follows:

- Problems the patient is aware of
- Problems the patient is unlikely to be aware of.

All the problems that can arise, either directly or indirectly, ultimately affect whether or not alignment can be maintained, and to what extent some level of misalignment has to be accepted. Furthermore, in the UK at least, in many clinical settings, the patient may also incur charges, e.g. for the replacement or repair of retainers.

Problems the patient is aware of

- Lack of fit
- Lack of alignment

Orthodontic Retainers and Removable Appliances: Principles of Design and Use, First Edition.
Friedy Luther and Zararna Nelson-Moon.
© 2013 Friedy Luther and Zararna Nelson-Moon. Published 2013 by Blackwell Publishing Ltd.

- Discomfort
- Lack of patient motivation
- Breakages

Lack of fit

If the patient has previously been appropriately instructed, they will hopefully realise themselves that their Hawley or vacuum-formed retainer (VFR) is not fitting properly. This can occur because, through wear and tear, the VFR plastic has 'given' a little or clasps have loosened up on a Hawley retainer (Figure 9.1). If this is the case, the patient will hopefully

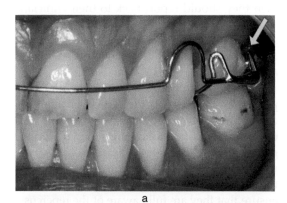

a

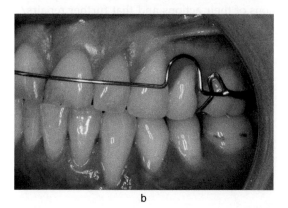

b

Figure 9.1 An Adams' clasp that has become loose (a, arrowed) through regular wear of a modified Hawley retainer. The labial bow has been soldered to the bridges of the Adams' clasps on this retainer. The clasp has been adjusted and tightened (b). (Photographs courtesy of Simon Littlewood and Carol Bentley.)

contact their orthodontist or dentist, i.e. whoever is responsible for monitoring and maintaining their retainer wear, so that adjustments or re-makes can be made as appropriate.

Lack of alignment

Of course, changes in alignment may occur through lack of fit, since a patient may fail to return in time for adjustments/re-makes. It is likely that any changes in alignment in these circumstances would have to be accepted unless an operator is either prepared to re-treat or there is scope to use a vacuum-formed active appliance (VFAA; see Chapter 11) to re-align very minor changes. However, the risk is ever present that changes in alignment can always re-appear in the future and it is simply not realistic for any patient to be on a potentially endless treadmill of re-treatment; nor would this be justifiable from the dental health perspective.

In contrast, minor changes in tooth position occurring over long periods of time may be less obvious to the patient as they see their teeth every day. It is not intended that patients wear their retainers full time forever. Therefore, nights-only or alternate-night wear can allow some tooth movement. Of course, patients may occasionally forget to wear their retainer too. These are the reasons why one cannot guarantee that there will never be any tooth movement – even when a patient is wearing a retainer (Figure 9.2) and regardless of whether a retainer is of the removable sort or bonded. The problems associated with bonded retainers are described below. Again, the main way of dealing with this problem is by explaining to the patient/parent/guardian at the initial consent stage what can (and cannot) be expected of treatment. Retainers may *minimise* tooth movement, but cannot be guaranteed to *eliminate* the possibility of all tooth movement.

Discomfort

Removable retainers may rub the sulcus or gingivae, particularly following initial fitting.

Most commonly for a lower Hawley this occurs in the lingual sulcus. Patients should be encouraged to continue wearing the retainer, but to return as soon as possible to have it eased. This provides the maximum chance of the operator being able to see the exact location of the problem, so trimming and easing can be carried out to greatest effect. Furthermore, continuing wear means that the risk of tooth movement is minimised.

For Hawley retainers, easing can easily be undertaken with a straight handpiece and an acrylic bur. For VFRs, rubbing or irritation is likely to occur against the gingivae. Easing of VFRs is described in Chapter 8.

Lack of patient motivation

If a patient fails to wear a retainer as instructed, there is probably little that can be done other than to warn them of the likely consequences of their actions, i.e. the teeth are likely to move out of position and this would have to be accepted.

Of course, lack of patient motivation may demonstrate itself in other forms, e.g. poor dental health maintenance or broken appliances. These problems will be dealt with elsewhere.

Breakages

If the patient notices any retainer breakage, then they should report back to their clinician as soon as possible for a repair or re-make as needed. Clearly, if an appliance is broken, it cannot maintain the alignment of the teeth appropriately (Figures 9.3 and 9.4).

It is important that the clinician treating the patient establishes whether the breakage has occurred simply through wear and tear (e.g. one breakage occurs following a long period of good wear) or through carelessness or lack of motivation. If the latter, a discussion should take place with the patient/parent/guardian to ensure that they are fully aware of the repercussions of their actions and that further repairs/

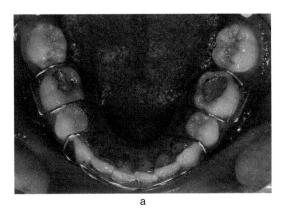

a

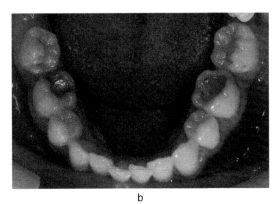

b

Figure 9.2 Example of minor tooth movement occuring despite reliable, alternate-night Hawley retainer wear. (a) With retainer; (b) without. These movements gradually became evident after about 2 years of regular retainer wear.

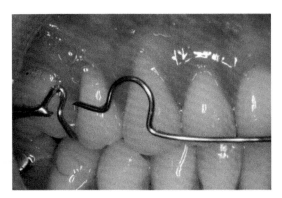

Figure 9.3 A labial bow breakage. The labial bow has fractured at its solder joint to the bridge of an Adams' clasp of a modified Hawley retainer. Clearly, alignment could be compromised until repair can be undertaken. (Photograph courtesy of Simon Littlewood.)

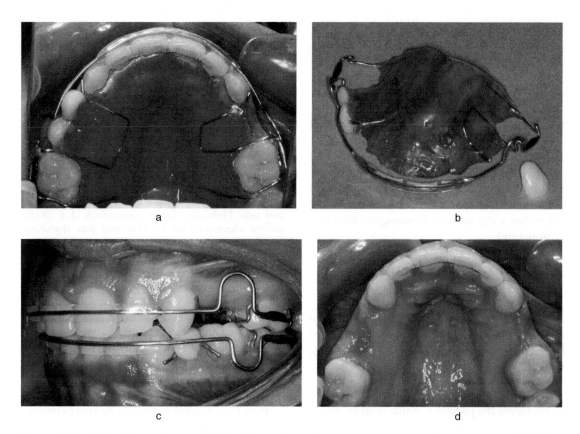

a   b

c   d

Figure 9.4 A Hawley retainer, modified with acrylic teeth, to maintain space and appearance until bridges or implants can be placed (a–d). In this case, a false tooth has fractured off the appliance (a–c). However, tooth movement into any spaces has been minimised, though not eliminated, due to use of a bonded retainer (d) and use of wire stops and clasp fly-overs (a–c). (Photographs courtesy of Simon Littlewood.)

re-makes cannot be guaranteed regardless of any other factors. In rare cases it may be necessary to terminate treatment (see below for a discussion of managing retention/treatment termination).

Problems the patient is unlikely to be aware of

Dental health: caries and periodontal problems

Removable retainers, as with any appliance in the mouth such as a partial denture or bridge, will automatically increase the oral bacterial load and plaque retention factors. Therefore, caries and periodontal disease are a greater risk in patients with retainers. This is true regardless of the fact that the appliance can and must be removed to allow oral hygiene measures to take place. However, this does not mean the patient's oral hygiene and care with diet (the latter from the caries point of view) will automatically be good.

Removable retainers, therefore, do have an advantage over fixed retainers in that they can be removed for cleaning. Despite this advantage however, it should not be assumed that dental health cannot be affected. Specifically, areas that can be especially affected are those that are hidden (or comparatively so) from the patient's view, e.g. palatal surfaces, upper incisors, upper and lower gingival margins. Once gingival swelling occurs, it becomes more feasible for plaque to build up sub-gingivally. These issues explain why regular follow-up by the responsible clinician is essential for proper and thorough oral hygiene and dental health assessment and re-inforcement of need for good oral hygiene. Ultimately however, should oral health not improve, then consideration may need to be given to terminating retention (see below for a discussion of managing retention termination).

Problems with bonded retainers and trouble-shooting

As with removable retainers, the problems that can arise with bonded retainers can be grouped in a similarly convenient and clinically realistic way:

- Problems the patient is aware of
- Problems the patient is unlikely to be aware of.

All the problems that can arise, either directly or indirectly, ultimately affect whether or not alignment can be maintained and to what extent some level of misalignment has to be accepted. *In the case of bonded retainers however, there is probably an increased risk that dental health could be compromised too.*

Problems the patient is aware of

- Lack of alignment
- Discomfort

Lack of alignment

Unfortunately, because the bonded retainer is always out of the patient's direct view, the patient is unlikely to realise that there is a problem until they notice a tooth or teeth are no longer aligned.

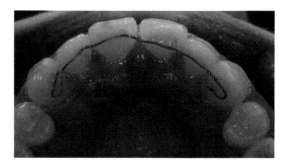

Figure 9.5   A bonded retainer demonstrating fracture and fraying of the multi-strand wire due to wear and tear. Note also the re-appearance of a small, midline diastema (due to wear and tear stretching the wire).

This will usually be caused by one or more of the following breakages indirectly causing lack of alignment.

- **A composite 'blob' debonds from the palatal or lingual surface of the tooth.** This may affect one or more composite bonds and, therefore, several teeth may be free to move. In our experience, this is the most common cause of retainer breakage. See Figure 8.5 for an example.

  Rarely, the patient may have heard a small 'crack' as the debond occurs or may detect a different 'feel' with their tongue. In these cases, the patient will hopefully return to have their bonded retainer checked and repaired as needed before any malalignment occurs.

- **Wire fracture.** In our experience, this is not very common, but if it does occur one or more teeth are free to move (Figure 9.5). Once again, the patient may be aware of a change in the 'feel' of their retainer when they run their tongue over it, but commonly the patient will be oblivious of any problem until some tooth movement occurs. However, to the supervising clinician it is usually obvious on examination that the wire has snapped. The exception may be when the broken ends of the wire remain lined up exactly with each other and there are no frayed ends to mark the spot.

- **Wire distortion.** Whilst we are unaware of any specific, detailed data, wire distortion on its own also seems to be a relatively uncommon problem. However, it is certainly more common when one or more composite blobs debond and the patient fails to notice this. In these circumstances, the length of free wire can then be very prone to distortion (as the patient continues with oral function) and this may render repair impossible.

Discomfort

Most patients seem to have few, if any, problems adapting to the presence of a bonded retainer. Therefore, it is unusual for patients to complain of any discomfort. If they do, the cause should be established as it is likely that there is a problem with the retainer. For example, a patient could complain of irritation/rubbing of the tongue if the wire has fractured or come away from the composite and is distorted. Another possibility is the multi-strand wire has started to unravel. If even one of the wires composing the multi-stranded wire snaps, this can present as a tiny spike that can cause significant tongue irritation out of all proportion to its size. Unfortunately, if any of these problems exist, there is no simple solution or repair that can be carried out. Depending on other factors, the only means of repairing the problem is to remove the entire retainer, make a new retainer and then rebond it into position. However, as discussed below, there are situations where re-making and rebonding is either contraindicated or impossible.

Problems the patient is unaware of

- Breakages: composite debond, wire fracture, wire distortion
- Wear and tear problems
- Dental health problems

- Increase in overbite
- Problems with rebonding

Breakages

- **Composite debond.** As noted above, the patient may notice that a composite blob has debonded, but, far more frequently, *the patient will be completely unaware of the problem*. This is because usually when debonds occur, there is only a minute gap between the composite and the surface of the tooth (see above). Not only can tooth movement occur, but plaque build up can also occur under the loose composite, leading to risk of caries.

  It is precisely because such debonds are likely to be invisible to the patient that good patient care demands regular review. Patients should not normally be discharged without follow-up being arranged, e.g. with their own dentist.

  In general, if a bonded retainer is placed, it is worth trying to see the patient at 3-month intervals for one or two visits. If all is well, review at 6-month intervals would then seem appropriate. However, if the patient suffers debonds or oral health problems, then, following any remedial action as needed, it is worth seeing the patient at shorter intervals until it is established whether or not they are able to proceed without any further problems developing.

- **Wire fracture.** This is usually obvious to the operator when they examine the patient, but as described above, the patient may well be entirely unaware of any problem with their retainer. The operator may miss a fracture when the broken ends of the wire remain lined up exactly with each other and there are no frayed ends to mark the spot. In order to detect this at follow-up, the operator should use a sharp probe and gently push the stretches of wire linking the teeth in case this type of break has occurred.

- **Wire distortion.** Again, this is usually obvious to the operator when they examine the patient, but the patient may well be entirely unaware of any problem with their retainer. Wire distortion without a wire break or any composite debonding can result in a tooth or teeth being actively moved out of position.

Wear and tear problems

Problems arising from wear and tear are little reported in the literature, perhaps because they tend to take place slowly as 'wear and tear' takes time to become apparent. There is still a dearth of good studies investigating and reporting on what happens to bonded retainers long term.

Examples of wear and tear problems that we have seen include spacing or diastemas re-opening despite an *intact* bonded retainer being in place. This is because the wire can stretch as a result of long-term bombardment by food and chewing activity. Wear marks may be seen, with the wire looking shiny or even flattened (Figure 9.6).

Composite may also be worn away and leave the wire exposed. Again, the retainer may be intact, but it is gradually being weakened.

Dental health problems

The main problems relate to the possibility of caries and/or periodontal problems. Most frequently, the patient will be entirely unaware of any problems as the retainer cannot be seen under direct vision. Of course, the other problem is that both diseases are usually painless in the initial stages and may only be slowly progressive. Studies to date suggest that these diseases are not really significant problems and that most patients will have few problems. However, this assumes that the studies are good enough to reflect the true situation. Unfortunately, this is probably not the case since studies undertaken around the world will reflect, to some extent at least, the healthcare systems present at the time. These may differ greatly from

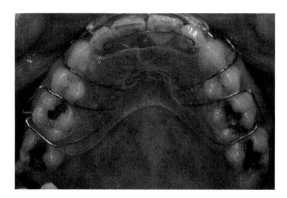

Figure 9.6 A patient's midline diastema is gradually re-appearing due to wear and tear of the retainer wire, resulting in the wire gradually stretching. The patient has been wearing the retainer for over 3 years. Note also the shiny areas on the wire, indicating the maximum areas of wear, e.g. directly behind the central incisors in the diastema region. The patient also wears an upper Hawley retainer due to their unfavourable lower lip position, which may move the upper incisors forward once more – a movement a bonded retainer could not prevent. This patient had suffered periodontal problems pre-treatment, but the need to maintain excellent oral hygiene post-treatment is evident here and clearly requires further attention.

country to country. This factor will influence the patient base and how it behaves. Furthermore, studies are inherently biased if they are only based on those patients willing to re-attend perhaps after many years. These patients may simply be those with the greatest interest in their own dental health and may, thus, represent a biased sample.

In general, due to the invisibility of the potential problems to the patient, it makes sense to see the patient at least every 6 months, at least initially. This allows not only dental health problems to be assessed, but also checks for breakages. Should dental disease be diagnosed, then the patient should obviously be informed and steps taken to support them so that the problem(s) can be treated (Figures 9.7 and 9.8 give examples of dental health problems associated with an upper and lower bonded retainer, respectively. Figure 9.8 also

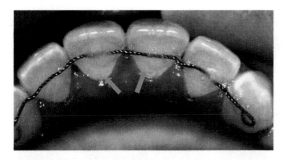

Figure 9.7 Example of demineralisation (arrowed) and gingival inflammation around an upper bonded retainer.

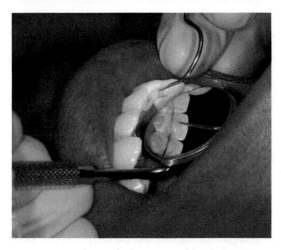

Figure 9.8 A bonded retainer with two problems: calculus build up around it and a debonded composite pad. Note how subtle the debond is: it can be detected by checking whether it is just possible to insert the tip of a dental probe lingual to it, as shown here.

highlights the subtle nature of debonds). Only if such help fails to address the problem should consideration be given to removing the retainer.

Another dental health problem that can arise is a bonded retainer becoming an active appliance. For example, if once bonded the retainer becomes badly distorted, e.g. the patient bites on something far too hard, directly onto the retainer wire, it is possible for the wire to then start moving the tooth or teeth through the labial plate. We are not aware of any formal case reports but, anecdotally, are aware of one

or two such episodes. Clearly, such problems may well directly affect a tooth's health and longevity.

Increase in overbite

It is easy to think that bonded retainers will stop all tooth movement. They do not. This is because failure rates reported in the literature are often quite high – even up to 40%. As noted above, once a breakage occurs, teeth are free to move (see Table 7.1).

One issue that can also arise with time, even when a bonded retainer remains intact, is the movement of the block of teeth to which the appliance is bonded. This movement is likely to be vertical. Therefore, even if, for example, the lower incisors formed an incomplete overbite at the time of bonding with the upper incisors, over time the bite may deepen, since teeth may still move either individually or *en bloc*. This deepening of the overbite may lead to significant problems. For example, when combined with wear and tear, the lower incisors, which may or may not have a bonded retainer in place, can still move as a unit and gradually wear down the upper arch palatal composite. Should the upper composite debond or wear down to the extent that composite replacement is required, then the overbite may have deepened by then such that composite replacement may be rendered impossible (see Figure 9.9 for details). If composite replacement is undertaken regardless of these circumstances, it is then very likely that the patient will not be able to tolerate such a build up since a lower incisor will now be biting hard on the new composite. Indeed, the lower teeth may bite off or through the composite, causing further breakage of the retainer.

Problems with rebonding

Each time a bracket or retainer has to be rebonded, the acid-etch process needs to be repeated. Phosphoric acid creates micropores

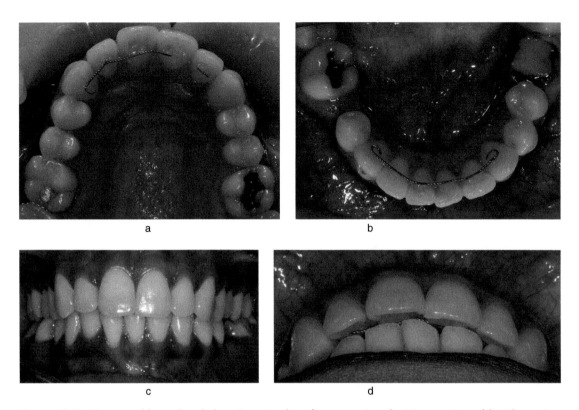

a   b

c   d

Figure 9.9 Upper and lower bonded retainers in place for approximately 10 years (a and b). The patient noticed slight movement of an upper incisor and felt something had changed on the upper retainer (a). It can be seen that through wear and tear, the upper bonded retainer has fractured between UL1 and UL2, and part of the wire has been lost. However, in addition more subtle changes can be seen (a): the composite has been worn from the occluding surface so that the retainer wire is now only held by composite beneath the wire (this is particularly obvious on UR1). As the overbite has increased with time, despite the lower bonded retainer, the proximity of the lower incisors to the upper bonded retainer is clear (c and d). This means that replacement of the upper bonded retainer is not simple, since removal of the old retainer and straight replacement with a new one is highly unlikely to be tolerated due to the increase in overbite that has ocurred and hence occlusal interferences. Therefore, it would either have to be removed and replaced with a removable retainer or further orthodontic movement is required to reduce the overbite once more, possibly combined with re-alignment of upper and lower incisors. If further treatment is pursued, the same cycle of events could be anticipated in future. Placement of a new retainer further gingivally is unlikely to be feasible in many cases since this may compromise gingival/periodontal health.

Note also that UR1 is no longer in total alignment with UL1 (a); likewise LR1 is no longer in complete alignment with LL1 (b), although no debonds or wire fractures have occurred here. This demonstrates that the wire can 'give' under wear and tear, allowing tooth movement to occur.

in the enamel surface. These pores allow composite tags to form a mechanical lock and thus allow the bonding process to be successful. Theoretically at least, this means that if the bracket or retainer has to be bonded back in more or less the same place, fewer pores will be available each time a rebond is required and each rebond could be weaker than the last. Of course, there is limited scope for rebonding the retainer into different, virgin enamel areas due to the occlusion as well as other practical restrictions. There is no specific evidence to confirm that repeated rebonding leads to a reduction in bond strength, but this is probably only because few studies have examined this possibility. The studies that have been undertaken are fairly inconclusive and have only assessed rebonding of brackets.

Bonded retainers: how to repair them

Once the clinical decision has been made to repair a debonded composite blob or pad, the following steps are advised:

1. Advise the patient how the repair is to be undertaken, but warn them that as composite is removed from the wire, the vibrations could loosen adjacent composite bonds. This is particularly true when the debond has occurred on the last standing tooth that was bonded.
2. Fit the patient, yourself and the nurse with safety spectacles.
3. Get ready a right-angled handpiece with a tungsten carbide composite-removing bur. Higher torque will help reduce the vibrations, not only from the patient's perspective, but also by helping to reduce the risk of adjacent debonds occurring. It will also remove the composite quicker.
4. It is essential that all composite at the debonded blob is removed. This includes any composite adhering to the wire and/or tooth. To achieve this most effectively, the tooth and composite should be blown dry prior to composite removal with the bur. Your nurse should supply high-speed suction to evacuate the dust generated by the composite removal, helping you to maintain clear vision and preventing dust obscuring your mirror.
5. Once a thin layer of composite is left on the archwire, e.g. 0.5–1-mm thick, it may be possible to 'nibble' it off using pliers, such as Weingart's, rather than continuing with a bur. These should be used to carefully press the composite against the wire, and it will then crumble away. However, great care is needed to avoid distorting the wire or allowing the composite fragments to shatter uncontrollably. Therefore, high-speed suction as the pliers are used is of great help.
6. You should now have a clean lingual or palatal tooth surface and a clean, intact wire with no composite adhering anywhere. It should be washed and dried with water, and the acid-etch procedure can then follow, ensuring full isolation of the tooth to allow a dry field.
7. Once the repair has been undertaken, check the occlusion with articulating paper and relieve as needed (see Chapter 8 and Figure 8.4). Check the inter-proximal contacts with floss. Again, clear the contacts as needed.

When repairs are not possible

It may not always be possible to repair damage to the bonded retainer. Examples include:

- Wire distorted
- Composite debonded and wire distorted
- Wire fracture
- Multi-stranded wire unravelling.

All of these circumstances will mean that the whole bonded retainer has to be removed and a decision made as to whether:

- A new bonded retainer can be placed
- Retention is to be stopped altogether
- The bonded retainers are to be replaced with a removable retainer.

The decision will be influenced by factors such as the:

- Cause of the problem and frequency of occurrence
- Feasibility of replacement with regard to the occlusion

- Patient's oral hygiene/dental health and general level of commitment to looking after their teeth and retainer.

No two cases are the same and each case has to be assessed individually. Therefore, the suggestions in this section can only highlight some of the factors that may require consideration.

An exception where total removal of the retainer may *not* be necessary can occur if the wire has simply fractured between the penultimate and last tooth in the line of bonded teeth, e.g. an upper canine-to-canine bonded retainer where the wire has fractured between an upper lateral and canine. In this situation it may be acceptable and possible to remove the composite and wire from the canine, and trim or smooth the end of the wire so it finishes at the upper lateral only. Whether or not this is an acceptable solution will depend on how important it is that the canine remains as part of the bonded retainer. For instance, if the canine was severely rotated prior to orthodontic treatment or if there was a large gap between the canine and lateral pre-treatment, the option may be less feasible than if the canine was merely included in the retainer as a convenient place to finish the retainer. This is due to the relapse tendency being greater for spacing and rotations.

Managing treatment termination and removal of retainers

There are occasions when a patient may simply wish to stop wearing their retainers and if the retainers are removable, that is easy enough for them to do. The clinician who carried out the patient's treatment should already have explained to the patient/parent/guardian, before treatment ever started and again in the lead up to retainers being placed, why retainers are used and what patients may expect to happen when retainers are no longer worn. That being

the case, the patient therefore makes an informed decision of their own – in which they accept the consequences of their own actions. That is, having stopped wearing the retainers, the teeth are more likely to move and if they do, this does not constitute a reason for re-treatment.

More difficult situations occur when patients fail to maintain adequate levels of dental care/co-operation, or sustain repeated breakages to their retainers or a breakage occurs which does not allow a simple repair to be a carried out.

In all these cases, much depends on what and how things have been discussed previously with the patient/parent/guardian and how their expectations have been previously managed. For example, if a patient is aware of the need to maintain good dental health and a careful diet, but fails in this regard on a number of occasions despite this being pointed out to them, it will be no great surprise to them if treatment or retention has to be stopped as problems arise, e.g caries.

It is difficult to give precise instructions about what to do in every situation, but some general principles or suggestions may help. It is important to be aware that serious confrontation can be avoided if it is apparent that the clinician is committed to helping patients and takes the time and trouble to explain things carefully, thoroughly and in a way the patient/parent/guardian can understand. It is helpful to relate the issues directly to the patient's own circumstances rather than speaking only in general, vague or theoretical terms.

1. Always explain and warn patients early on (before treatment starts) of what they can/cannot expect from treatment, and what eventualities they are likely to have to consider along the way. Document these discussions.
2. Monitor, document and act on issues that arise in treatment, explaining to the patient/parent/guardian what the issue is and what the consequences can be if nothing is done. For example, monitor oral hygiene or break-

ages and provide the patient with information and help as to how to overcome the problem. Explain what the consequences can be if nothing is done or the matter not corrected.

3. If the problems recur and the patient fails to respond adequately to the advice or help offered, then this should be explained to the patient/parent/guardian and at that point it may be appropriate to advise them that treatment termination may now need to be considered if things do not improve quickly. Ensure you explain again what the consequences will be and what the patient will have to accept if treatment has to be terminated. Document this too and consider a follow-up letter explaining and re-iterating this.

4. If the matter continues, then explain why it is now necessary to terminate treatment and again explain what the consequences will be.

By taking this sort of approach, we have generally found that far from the situation being confrontational, the patient/parent/guardian accepts what may turn out to be an inevitable conclusion for them. However, the crucial points are that the patient/parent/guardian is made aware of:

- What the issue was
- The problems caused by the issue
- The consequences for the patient if retention has to be terminated
- The clinician has offered support to help correct the problem, even though on this occasion the patient has not been able to do so.

What consequences need to be explained to the patient when retainers have to be stopped?

- Re-iterate that teeth have a tendency to move throughout life and it is common to see mild increases in crowding in untreated individuals. So without retainers, the teeth will be more likely to move throughout the patient's adult life. However, this does not necessarily mean a return to the original malocclusion, although it may well do if a mild malocclusion has been treated.
- Such movement, if it occurs, will have to be accepted; re-treatment would not normally be considered.
- It is better to accept the above rather than hang on to straighter teeth that are diseased and whose prognosis is, or will be, compromised.
- No retainer can guarantee that no tooth movement will ever arise.

In the case of a patient who has multiple, persistent and frequent breakages, it is not normally feasible to consistently and continuously provide all the repairs required. Indeed, the patient is unlikely to be able to attend frequently enough for repairs to be carried out so rapidly that all tooth movement is prevented. Therefore, treatment termination in this situation is likely to be the consequence, as the likely tooth movement will prevent repair.

Rarely, a patient may have undergone fixed appliance therapy to re-align teeth that have drifted severely due to periodontal disease. Orthodontic treatment is only undertaken if and when the periodontal disease has been *fully controlled*. Following such treatment, bonded retainers usually have to be placed, but there then *has* to be a lifelong commitment by the patient to maintain excellent dental health if they wish retention to continue. This normally means ongoing, lifelong, regular and possibly frequent periodontal support. Should this not be the case for whatever reason, then the likelihood is that the patient has to be counselled that the retainer be removed and any relapse (which is likely to be very significant) accepted. If the patient refuses to allow the retainer to be removed, then it must be very clearly explained what the consequences of their decision may be. Of course, this includes the possibility of tooth loss. This should be clearly documented in the notes.

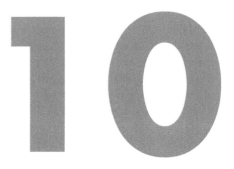

Removable Appliances for the Postgraduate in Specialist Orthodontic Training

This chapter will give an overview of the types of removable appliances that may be used as part of the definitive treatment for some of the more severe malocclusions. The treatment of these malocclusions and the use of the appliances discussed should not be undertaken without the appropriate theoretical knowledge and practical experience. Therefore, this treatment is really the preserve of the specialist orthodontist or those treating patients under the close supervision of a specialist orthodontist.

However, it is hoped that this chapter will serve as a useful source of basic information for those just starting on their postgraduate training, and also provide some direction for further reading and learning for those who are less experienced, but wish to develop their knowledge further.

The chapter will be divided into three sections covering:

* Removable appliances for correcting excessive positive overjets

* Removable appliances and their role in correcting Class II molar relationships
* Removable appliances for correcting reverse overjets.

> **Learning outcomes**
>
> At the end of this chapter you will be able to:
>
> * List several appliances that may be used for the correction of excessive positive and negative overjets and molar relationships
> * Describe the effects that the appliances may have on the dentition and facial skeleton, including the potential hazards of headgear wear
> * Realise the necessity for significant theoretical knowledge and supervised practical experience before using these appliances without direct supervision by an appropriately trained person

Orthodontic Retainers and Removable Appliances: Principles of Design and Use, First Edition.
Friedy Luther and Zararna Nelson-Moon.
© 2013 Friedy Luther and Zararna Nelson-Moon. Published 2013 by Blackwell Publishing Ltd.

Removable appliances for correcting excessive positive overjet

Removable appliances for the correction of excessive positive overjet are commonly referred to as functional appliances in the UK. However, they are also known as orthopaedic or growth modification devices because of their perceived effect on maxillary and mandibular growth.

The term 'functional' appliance derives from the initial use of these appliances, which aimed to alter the function of the mandible and its musculature by forcing the patient to posture the mandible forward, so reducing the overjet. The stretching of the muscles caused by this was thought to encourage growth of the mandible.

Certainly, growth of the mandible does occur at the condyles with some remodelling of the glenoid fossa. It is possible to see a change in shape and length of the condyles between pre-treatment and post-functional lateral skull radiographs. Growth of the condyles is required to maintain the mandible in the 'postured' position as, once the functional appliance is withdrawn, any change in position of the mandible that was due to 'training' of the masticatory muscles will become apparent very quickly as the muscles 'de-train' and the mandible returns to its original position. However, it is now thought that functional appliances accelerate and redirect the growth of the mandible, rather than increase its growth beyond what has been genetically predetermined.

Historically, functional appliances were used in the treatment of Class II division 1 malocclusions where the upper and lower arches were well aligned, the upper incisors were proclined and there was a Class II skeletal pattern. However, this was in the days when functional appliances were used in isolation to treat Class II division 1 malocclusions and their use was not followed by a course of fixed appliance treatment. These days, the majority of patients have fixed appliance treatment following an initial phase with a functional appliance to correct the overjet and molar relationship. Crowding and alignment of the teeth can then be corrected during the phase of fixed appliance treatment, with or without extractions of permanent teeth. Furthermore, the residual lateral open bites can be closed. Occasionally, these do not close spontaneously.

A wealth of literature, both in textbooks and journal articles, has been published on the use of and theory behind functional appliances. Unfortunately, it is not possible to draw firm conclusions from many of the older research papers as the methods and statistical analyses are flawed. However, it is imperative that the clinician has a good background knowledge of functional appliances before embarking on any such treatments, as inappropriate/inaccurate provision, design and instructions on wear can have a very deleterious effect on the patient's malocclusion, facial appearance, treatment time, expectations and co-operation.

Effects of functional appliances

A well-worn functional appliance will, relatively rapidly in a growing individual, change the molar relationship and reduce the overjet and overbite. All of these changes are usually desired, but functional appliances also produce some changes that are not always advantageous, e.g. increase in the lower anterior face height and proclination of the lower incisors.

The effects of the use of functional appliances on the correction of a Class II division 1 malocclusion are both dental (70%) and, generally to a far lesser extent, skeletal (30%). A more recent multicentre randomized controlled trial has indicated that these figures vary with the parameter being measured (O'Brien et al., 2003). In this study, 73% of overjet reduction and 59% of molar correction was dental. However, the authors reported significant individual variation in the response to functional appliance therapy and, clinically, variation in response is what is typically seen.

Dental effects

- Retroclination of the upper labial segment (ULS)
- Proclination of the lower labial segment (LLS)

Leading to:

- Reduction in overjet
- Reduction in overbite
- Mesial movement of lower molars
- Distal tipping of upper molars.

Skeletal effects

These are generally far less predictable than the dental effects, but include:

- Acceleration of mandibular growth
- Retardation of maxillary growth
- Remodelling of the condyle
- Remodelling of the glenoid fossa
- Increase in lower anterior face height.

Figures 10.1 and 10.2 show the pre- and post-treatment intra- and extra-oral clinical photographs, respectively, of a patient who underwent 6 months of treatment with a functional appliance (Twin Block). It is apparent that the appliance has corrected the overjet and molar relationship, but has had a lesser effect on the skeletal pattern, although there has been a beneficial increase in lower anterior face height.

Clark Twin Block

This appliance was introduced by William J. Clark, a specialist orthodontic practitioner working in Scotland, in the 1980s (Clark, 1982). In the last 30 years it has become the most popular functional appliance to be used by orthodontists in the world. Its popularity has arisen due to the perceived ease of wear of this appliance, which comes as separate upper and lower blocks worn as a pair (twin blocks), compared to the more traditional functional appliances, which are fabricated as a single appliance (monobloc).

Indications

- Class II malocclusion with mild/moderate Class II skeletal pattern
- Class II molar relationship
- Increased overjet
- Proclined upper incisors
- Lower incisors that are not already excessively proclined
- Reduced or average vertical proportions

Contra-indications

- Significant anterior open bite
- Significantly increased vertical proportions
- Excessively proclined lower incisors

Design features (Figures 10.3 and 10.4)

Since its introduction, there have been a number of designs and modifications of the Twin Block, but one of the most frequently used designs is described below.

Active:

Midline expansion screw.
Posterior acrylic blocks.
±Labial bow on ULS.

Retention:

Adams' clasps on all four first permanent molars and all four first premolar teeth.
Ball-ended clasps on lower incisor teeth.
Labial bow on ULS.

Anchorage: Reciprocal anchorage using posterior acrylic blocks and the mesialising effect on the lower arch and the distalising effect on the upper arch.

Baseplate: Midline split in upper appliance to allow expansion.

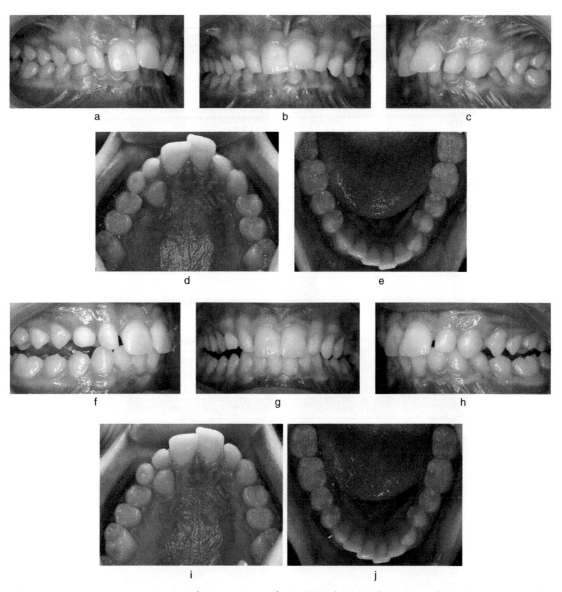

Figure 10.1   Pre-treatment (a–e) and post-treatment (f–j) intra-oral views of a patient who underwent 6 months of functional appliance (Twin Block) treatment. Note the correction of the incisor and molar relationship to Class I. Also note the lateral open bites in the post-treatment photographs caused by the posterior biteblocks on the Twin Block appliance. Fixed appliances will now be needed to complete treatment.

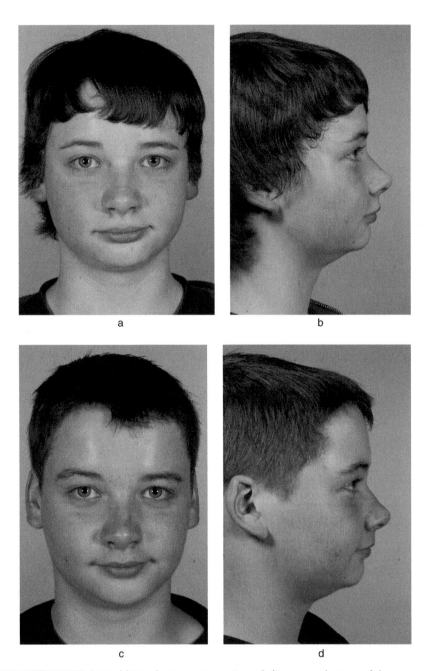

a

b

c

d

Figure 10.2   Pre-treatment (a and b) and post-treatment (c and d) extra-oral views of the same patient as in Figure 10.1, treated for 6 months with a functional appliance. Note that there has been less correction of the Class II skeletal discrepancy than there has of the Class II malocclusion (Figure 10.1). There has been a beneficial post-treatment increase in lower anterior face height and a reduction in depth of the labio-mental fold.

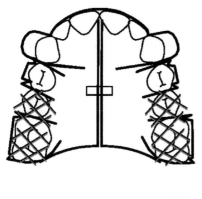

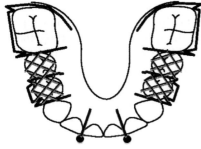

Please construct a Clark Twin Block:

1. Midline expansion screw

2. Adams' clasps UR64, UL46, LL64, LR46 – 0.7 mm hard ss wire

3. Labial bow UR321, UL123 – 0.7 mm hard ss wire

4. Ball-ended clasps LR21, LL12

5. Midline split in baseplate as indicated

6. Posterior bite blocks: 45° slope and 7 mm height

Figure 10.3 Laboratory prescription for a Twin Block appliance to reduce the overjet and correct the Class II molar relationship.

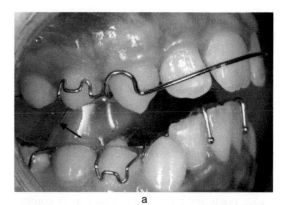

a

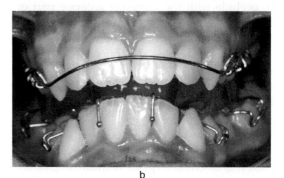

b

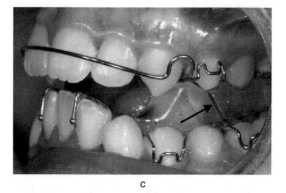

c

Figure 10.4 Intra-oral views (a–c) of a Twin Block *in situ*; prescription as indicated in Figure 10.3. Note the 45° slope of the upper and lower posterior bite-blocks (arrowed in a and c) as they interlock to keep the mandible in a postured position.

Posterior acrylic blocks with mesial aspect of upper block and distal aspect of lower block angulated at 45°.

Retention is provided by the Adams' clasps, ball-ended clasps and labial bow. However, if the upper incisors are excessively proclined and spaced, the labial bow can be converted into an active component (see Chapter 4). The midline expansion screw is included as posterior crossbites are often induced as the mandible is positioned more anteriorly and the wider posterior part of the lower arch comes to occlude with the narrower anterior part of the upper arch.

The 'active' part of the Twin Block appliance is the acrylic blocks. These were originally designed with a 45° slope on the anterior of the upper block and the posterior of the lower block. As the patient postures forward, the slope on the blocks causes them to interlock, keeping the mandible in the postured position.

If the second permanent molars are erupted, then it is essential to place occlusal stops over these teeth to prevent them from over-erupting. If unerupted, they should be incorporated as soon as they erupt.

Construction

Assuming high-quality impressions, the most important record to collect in order to construct a Twin Block, or any other functional appliance, is the postured bite registration. Although there are a number of different ways of doing this, the principles remain the same:

- The patient should be asked to posture the mandible as far forward as they can achieve comfortably, ideally in an edge-to-edge incisor relationship.
- Assuming that there is no mandibular displacement from the retruded contact position (RCP) into the inter-cuspal position (ICP), care must be taken to ensure that the upper and lower dental centre-line relationship is not altered as the mandible is pos-

tured, as a mandibular asymmetry can be induced if the mandible is postured more on one side than the other.

The postured bite may be recorded with either a softened horse-shoe of bite-registration wax at the required thickness or a ProJet® bite-fork, following the manufacturer's instructions.

Fitting the appliance

All the principles discussed in Chapter 4 are pertinent to the fitting of functional appliances: checking the appliance before fitting; the advice that should be given to the patient prior to fitting; the way in which the fit of the appliance is checked by the operator, and the adjustments required to increase the retention of the appliance. It is assumed that the reader is already familiar with the content of Chapter 4.

The upper part of the Twin Block should be fitted first, and then removed whilst the lower part of the Twin Block is fitted. Once both parts are fitting well and are retentive, they should both be placed in the patient's mouth, upper first followed by the lower, and the patient should be advised to posture the mandible forward until the lower block slides up in front of the upper block and is held in this postured position. The patient should be advised that this is the position that they must always bite in when the appliance is in place, because otherwise the appliance will not work. It helps to provide lots of positive encouragement by showing the patient and the parent that, in the postured position, the top teeth no longer stick out and it is easier to get the lower lip in front of them.

It is essential that the overjet, molar relationship and canine relationship are measured without the appliance in place and with the mandible in its most retruded position. It is also essential to check that there is sufficient activation with the appliance in place and that the patient's mandible is being held in at least a Class I relationship, preferably edge-to-edge.

Instructions/advice to patient/parent/guardian

The generic advice for the wear of removable appliances detailed in Chapter 4 applies to functional appliances as well, although with some additional information:

- The patient should be warned that not only will the teeth feel uncomfortable for a few days, but the sides of the face will be sore as well. This soreness is due to the stretching of the masseter muscle as the mandible is postured and will continue until the fibres of the masseter muscle have increased in length, which takes a few days. It is important to emphasise to the patient and parent that the soreness will only resolve if the appliance is worn well as the 'muscles need to get used to the new position'. It will not resolve if the appliance is continuously taken in and out.
- Although difficult, it is possible for the patient to eat with the Twin Block in place and they should be actively encouraged to wear it for eating. All other functional appliances, which are fabricated as a single block, have to be removed for eating.

Follow-up appointments

The patient should be reviewed every 6–8 weeks whilst the Twin Block is being worn full-time. Chapter 5 details the features that should be checked in all patients wearing removable appliances. However, there are a number of key additional measurements to record if the patient is wearing a functional appliance:

- The overjet, molar relationship and canine relationship should be measured and re-corded at every visit. If the patient has been wearing the appliance well, their masticatory musculature will have adapted to the postured position of the mandible and, even

without the appliance in place, the patient will tend to bite in the postured position. This may not be the true, anatomical position of the mandible and the clinician needs to develop a reliable method of ensuring that the patient is in the RCP when the measurements are taken.
- The transverse relationship should also be monitored at every visit and, if it becomes apparent that a posterior crossbite is developing, the patient should be instructed to start turning the midline expansion screw by a ¼ turn on a weekly basis (see Chapter 4).

With the standard design of appliance, you can expect to see an overjet reduction of at least 3 mm and change in molar relationship of at least ¼ unit after the first two follow-up visits. The progress tends to slow down as the mandible comes forward and the activation of the appliance becomes less.

If the overjet has only reduced by 1 mm, or not at all, then either the appliance is not active because the postured bite has not been taken accurately or, more likely, the patient is not wearing the appliance as instructed; either for insufficient hours or posturing incorrectly with the appliance in place. In this situation, the patient needs to be given lots of positive encouragement and an (easily achievable) target can be set to provide some focus for the patient in order to encourage them to increase the hours of wear. A reduction in overjet of 3 mm should be an easy target to achieve if the patient wears the appliance as instructed. If they are posturing incorrectly, then the patient must be re-instructed/ re-educated. Either way, the parents should, of course, be included in any discussions so that they can be informed of any problems and help to assess and monitor wear at home.

If the patient is unable to achieve the necessary hours of wear (24 hours a day except for the essential oral hygiene measures; contact sports; swimming, and eating if necessary) within two to three visits and despite encouragement, then consideration needs to be given to terminating treatment. Treatment that is not progressing satisfactorily should not be allowed to drag on since the risks of treatment do not go away and complications, if they do occur, may compromise any future treatment. Furthermore, patient co-operation may be burnt out by a prolonged, but unsuccessful, course of treatment.

Managing the end of the functional appliance treatment and retention

The functional appliance should be worn full-time until the molar relationship is super-Class I and the overjet has been reduced to 1 mm. This allows for the inevitable small amount of relapse that occurs once the appliance stops being worn.

As with all appliances that have posterior capping (when worn properly), Twin Blocks induce a lateral open bite. There are a number of ways of managing the withdrawal of the appliance:

- The acrylic blocks can be removed, apart from the most anterior part of the upper block and the most distal part of the lower block, which must be retained in order to maintain the postured bite. The appliance can then continue to be worn full-time, especially if the midline screw has been activated to expand the upper arch.
- If expansion has not been required, or was completed more than 3 months previously, then the appliance can be worn on a part-time basis – 12 hours in and 12 hours out. These 12 hours usually equate to wearing the appliance in the evenings and when in bed.

Either of these regimes should be continued for 3 months and then the position of the teeth re-measured to check that there has not been any significant relapse. Although a 1- or 2-mm increase in overjet is to be expected, any increase more than this is concerning and may indicate that the overjet measurements have been made with the mandible in a postured position rather than the RCP. Once the appli-

ance is being worn part-time, any posturing becomes apparent as the musculature de-programmes.

Assuming minimal relapse, up-to-date records should be taken to enable the fixed appliance phase of treatment to be planned.

Variations in the standard design

The Twin Block is a very adaptable appliance and a number of modifications can be made in order to customise the appliance for each individual malocclusion.

Other *active* components may be added, e.g. Z-springs to procline palatally positioned upper lateral incisors. This has the benefit of ensuring that the lateral incisors do not hinder the forward movement of the mandible, nor will they end up in a crossbite at the end of the functional phase of treatment (Figure 10.5).

In patients in whom the ULS is upright, rather than proclined, or the upper anterior teeth have been previously traumatised, it is possible to leave the labial bow off the design of the appliance. This modification will reduce the speed of overjet reduction, but will not affect the speed of molar relationship correction (Figure 10.5).

All functional appliances procline the lower incisors, but it is possible to reduce this a little by placing acrylic capping over the lower incisor teeth. This makes the appliance more difficult to wear and, especially, to eat with. Again, overjet reduction and molar correction will be slower, as the reduction in proclination of the lower incisors will prevent the lower molars from moving mesially so quickly. In essence, the change in overjet and molar relationship should, theoretically at least, be more skeletal than dental (Figure 10.6).

Other functional appliances

Although the Twin Block appliance is the most popular functional appliance, there are circumstances when the use of another functional appliance should be considered. The construc-

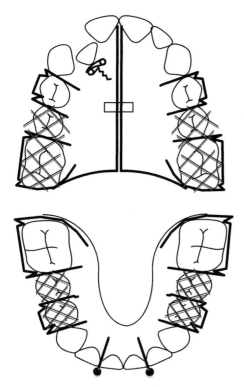

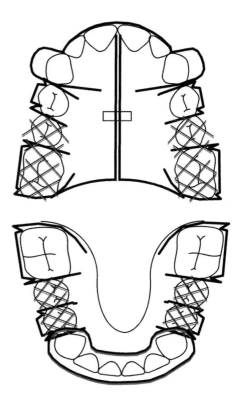

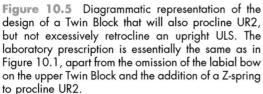

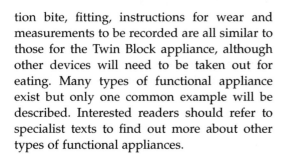

Figure 10.5 Diagrammatic representation of the design of a Twin Block that will also procline UR2, but not excessively retrocline an upright ULS. The laboratory prescription is essentially the same as in Figure 10.1, apart from the omission of the labial bow on the upper Twin Block and the addition of a Z-spring to procline UR2.

Figure 10.6 Diagrammatic representation of the design of a Twin Block that aims to reduce the amount of proclination of the LLS that occurs during correction of a Class II division 1 malocclusion. The ball-ended clasps (Figures 10.1 and 10.2) have been replaced with acrylic capping for the LLS.

tion bite, fitting, instructions for wear and measurements to be recorded are all similar to those for the Twin Block appliance, although other devices will need to be taken out for eating. Many types of functional appliance exist but only one common example will be described. Interested readers should refer to specialist texts to find out more about other types of functional appliances.

Medium opening activator

This appliance is fabricated as a single block and consists of retention provided by Adams' clasps on the upper first permanent molars (±

first premolars). There is a labial bow around the upper anterior segment and the mandible is held in the postured position by asking the patient to posture forward so that the lower incisors bite into the acrylic capping. This acrylic capping over the lower incisors is connected to the upper part of the appliance by two acrylic rods (Figure 10.7).

This appliance is useful for patients with very deep overbites and reduced lower anterior face height as the design leaves the lower posterior teeth completely free to erupt. However, it does not allow the upper arch to be expanded at the same time as the overjet correction.

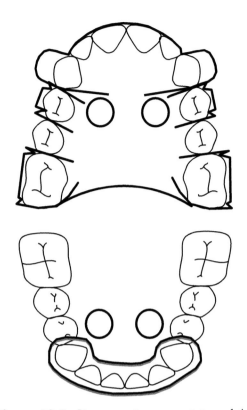

Figure 10.7 Diagrammatic representation of the design for a medium opening activator (MOA) to correct a Class II incisor and molar relationship. The appliance is retained in the mouth using Adams' clasps on the upper first permanent molars and upper first premolars, and the patient postures the mandible so that the lower incisors are positioned in the acrylic capping.

The retention period is achieved by the patient wearing the appliance on a part-time basis, 12 hours in and 12 hours out.

Removable appliances and their role in correcting molar relationships

The correction of molar relationships usually refers to the distalisation of the upper molars to create a Class I molar relationship. However, the change in molar relationship is also aided by the restraint of maxillary growth provided by the use of headgear. The use of a removable appliance with/without headgear support is a useful adjunct to fixed appliance therapy and may be carried out in the late mixed dentition. However, the change in molar relationship following exfoliation of the primary molars must always be taken into consideration during the treatment planning stage. It is also significantly easier for a patient to wear headgear with a removable appliance, because the appliance may be taken out of the mouth to allow the headgear facebow to be fitted to tubes soldered to the bridge of the Adams' clasps on the molars. Alternatively, tubes may be embedded into posterior capping.

The main types of appliances used to correct the molar relationship by distalising the upper molars are those to which headgear may be attached, e.g. an 'en masse' appliance; those used in conjunction with headgear attached to molar bands, e.g. a 'Nudger' appliance; and those with screws to distalise molars unilaterally, with or without headgear support.

Although each appliance has its own indications and contra-indications, the main consideration must be that it is very difficult to distalise upper molars by more than half a unit (i.e. from ½ unit Class II to Class I), even with the advent of temporary anchorage devices such as implants and mini-screws, especially if the second permanent molars are present.

The functional appliance is the main type of appliance for correcting the molar relationship by encouraging mesial movement of the lower molars. The change in molar relationship is brought about by distal tipping of the upper molars, mesial movement of the lower molars, encouragement of mandibular growth and restraint of maxillary growth. An appliance that is worn well is able to correct a molar relationship by at least one full unit, i.e. from a full unit Class II to Class I, although great care needs to be taken to avoid excessive proclination of the lower incisors (refer to previous section).

En masse appliance

This appliance consists of a URA with a midline expansion screw and headgear tubes soldered to the bridges of the Adams' clasps on the first permanent molar teeth. Although the original design of this appliance did not incorporate a biteplane of any description, our opinion is that incorporating posterior capping serves to disengage the occlusion and aid distal movement. Of course, if the overbite is already increased, then an anterior biteplane may be included instead of posterior capping. If the appliance is only required to be worn at the same time as the headgear, then an integral facebow may be incorporated into the appliance, which aids safety (see below).

Indications

* Distalisation of the upper molars by the same amount bilaterally when expansion of the upper arch is also required

Contra-indications

* Class I or Class III incisor relationships on Class III skeletal bases

Rationale: Headgear should not be used in these cases because of its effect on restricting the growth of the maxilla.

Design features (Figure 10.8)

Active: Midline expansion screw, headgear.

Retention: Adam's clasps on the upper first permanent molars (0.7 mm hard ss wire) and on the upper first premolars (0.7 mm wire) or upper first primary molars (0.6 mm wire).

Extra-oral traction (EOT) tubes soldered to the bridge of clasps on the upper first permanent molars.

Anchorage: Reciprocal: both sides of the arch will move equally in a buccal direction.

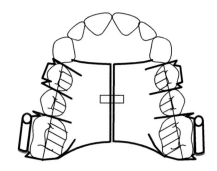

Please construct an upper removable appliance to expand the upper arch and aid molar distalisation:

1. Midline expansion screw

2. Adams' clasps UR6, UL6 – 0.7 mm hard ss wire

3. Adams' clasps UR4, UL4 – 0.7 mm hard ss wire

4. EOT tubes soldered to bridges of clasps on UR6, UL6

5. ½ occlusal coverage posterior capping

6. Midline split in baseplate as indicated

7. Baseplate saddled as indicated

Figure 10.8 Laboratory prescription for an 'en masse' URA to distalise the upper first permanent molars, in conjunction with extra-oral traction (EOT) , and expand the upper arch.

Baseplate: Midline split to allow expansion.

Half-occlusal coverage posterior capping to disengage occlusion and allow free movement of upper teeth:

* Because of occlusal interferences between the maxillary and mandibular teeth, failure to disclude the teeth in a well inter-digitated occlusion often results in concomitant expansion of the lower arch, with no correction of the transverse discrepancy between the two
* Posterior capping will encourage the incisors to erupt and so will increase the overbite. If the overbite is already increased and a further increase is contraindicated, then a

flat anterior biteplane may be included instead of posterior capping

Fitting the appliance

Refer to Chapter 4 for detailed instructions on the fitting of the removable appliance.

The fitting of headgear is not covered in this textbook. In our opinion, headgear should only be fitted by those who have undergone appropriate training in the theory and practice of headgear use. This type of training is provided on postgraduate courses.

Activation

Refer to Chapter 4 for detailed instructions on the activation of this type of appliance.

Nudger appliance

The Nudger is a URA used in conjunction with headgear attached to molar bands. It consists of Adams' clasps on the upper first premolar teeth, palatal finger springs mesial to the first permanent molars in 0.6 mm hard ss wire and a Southend clasp around the upper central incisors. A flat anterior biteplane is also included, which will decrease an increased overbite and, because it discludes the posterior teeth, helps with distal movement. The Nudger appliance should be worn full-time, even though the headgear will only be worn for 12–14 hours per day. The Nudger appliance should *not* be used to distalise upper first permanent molars without the use of headgear because of the effects of anchorage loss (see below).

It is important to note that the impression for the working model must be taken after the molar bands have been cemented in place.

Indications

* When asymmetric molar movement is required
* When the patient also has a deep overbite

Contra-indications

* The patient does not have any suitable teeth to retain the appliance, e.g. the first premolar teeth have not erupted yet or have already been extracted
* The patient refuses to wear headgear

Design features (Figures 10.9 and 10.10)

Active: Palatal finger springs on UR6, UL6 (0.6 mm hard ss wire).

Retention: Adams' clasps on UR4, UL4 (0.7 mm wire).
Southend clasp on UR1, UL1 (0.7 mm hard ss wire).

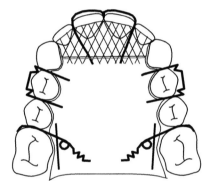

Please construct an upper removable appliance (Nudger) to aid with molar distalisation:

1. Palatal finger springs UR6, UL6 – 0.6 mm hard ss wire, boxed and guarded

2. Adams' clasps UR4, UL4 – 0.7 mm hard ss wire

3. Southend clasp UR1, UL1 – 0.7 mm hard ss wire

4. Flat anterior bite plane – please extend posteriorly by 8 mm (OJ 5 mm) and cover 2/3 of the height of the upper central incisor crowns

5. Please remove acrylic collets from distal of upper second premolars and upper first molars

Figure 10.9 Laboratory prescription for a 'Nudger' appliance to aid distal movement of the upper first permanent molars by extra-oral traction.

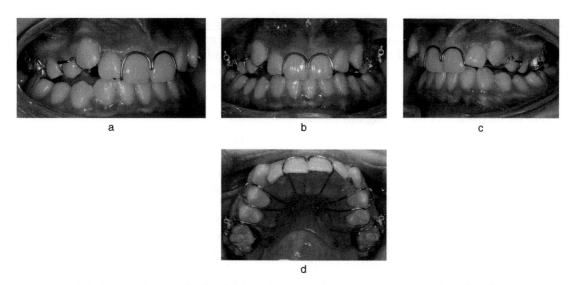

Figure 10.10 Intra-oral views of a 'Nudger' appliance *in situ*. Note the position of the palatal finger springs to aid molar distalisation (arrowed in a and c). The finger spring on UR6 is lying in the correct position (a and d), but the finger spring on UL6 (c and d) needs to be repositioned so that in lies mesial to UL6. In its current position, it is not active. Also note the presence of a flat anterior biteplane (FABP) (d) which has caused the upper and lower posterior teeth to become slightly separated (a–c), aiding distal movement of the upper buccal segments.

Anchorage: The effect of moving the first molars distally with the finger springs is to move the rest of the dentition mesially, potentially increasing the overjet. The headgear acts as the main distalisation force, with the finger springs acting as little more than retainers during the day when the headgear is not being worn. The Nudger appliance should *never* be used without headgear.

Baseplate: Flat anterior biteplane.

Boxed and guarded around finger springs.

The collets of acrylic should be removed from distal to the molars and second premolars to allow distal movement of these teeth.

Fitting of the appliance

The fitting of this appliance is little different from other appliances with flat anterior biteplanes and palatal finger springs (refer to the relevant sections in Chapter 4 for FABP and for finger springs).

Activation

Activation of the finger springs should follow the guidance given in Chapter 4 and aim to activate the springs by one-third of the mesio-distal width of the molar. However, if more distalisation is required on one side than on the other, the activation on the tooth that has less far to move should be reduced. The activation on the tooth that has to move further should not be increased beyond the recommended amount.

URA with expansion screw for distalisation

The appliance shown in Figure 3.6 can also be used with headgear to support the anchorage attached via tubes soldered to the bridge of the Adams' clasps on the molars. Activation of the screw supplies the force to distalise the molar, but as the equal and opposite response from the anchor teeth would be mesial movement, headgear worn for 10–12 hours per day can be a very useful method of preventing this mesial movement from occurring.

Headgear safety (Figure 10.11)

All headgear has to be provided with safety modifications because of the rare but potentially catastrophic effects that an accident with headgear can have on the patient. The inter-molar width is the same as the inter-pupillary width. Therefore, unless precautions are taken to prevent the facebow coming out of the mouth and/or the head cap acting as a catapult, serious damage to the eyes may result. This has

caused a number of unfortunate patients to go blind in the past (Booth-Mason and Birnie, 1988).

All manufacturers of headgear components now produce products that have been modified to comply with the safety requirements. These include:

* Locking facebows (that cannot be accidentally removed from molar tubes)
* Facebows that protect the 'sharp' end and reduce the risk of a penetrating injury
* Facebows that are inserted from behind the tube and so need to be taken out backward, rather than pulled out in a forward direction
* Snap-away head caps that prevent the head cap acting like a catapult
* Masel safety straps that are inelastic and prevent the facebow ends coming out of the patient's mouth.

It is imperative that the safety features and reasons for always using them are explained and demonstrated to the patient and parent. Should an eye injury with headgear occur or be suspected, the patient should be advised to attend Accident and Emergency immediately and seek an urgent ophthalmic opinion.

Other types of removable appliances for correcting reverse overjets

For the purpose of this chapter, a reverse overjet is defined as all four upper incisor teeth being in crossbite with the lower incisors. Removable appliances alone are rarely used for the definitive correction of reverse overjets. This type of malocclusion is usually associated with a Class III skeletal pattern and extreme caution needs to be applied when treating such cases because of the likelihood of further deterioration of the malocclusion during the adolescent growth spurt, especially in boys. The use of fixed appliances, even if a removable appliance has been

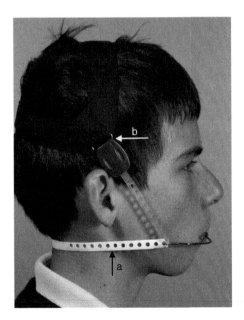

Figure 10.11 Extra-oral views of a patient wearing high-pull headgear. The safety features displayed include the Masel safety strap (a) and the snap-away feature on the head cap (b). The facebow is also designed to protect the 'sharp' end (not shown).

used as an interceptive measure, is required in the vast majority of cases.

Treatment planning and the consent to treatment of these cases are complex and the mechanics of treatment often demanding on the patient and orthodontist. Treatment of malocclusions of this type should be the preserve of the specialist orthodontist with the appropriate level of postgraduate training.

Indications

There are only a very small number of indications for removable appliances in patients with reverse overjets. These include:

- Young patients aged approximately 8 years old, with a hypoplastic/retrognathic maxilla
- Patients with severe hypodontia in whom the appliance is being used to support the anchorage.

In both of the above situations, the skeletal discrepancy should lie with the maxilla, with only a very mild prognathia of the mandible. Also, the overbite should be average, or preferably increased, because the mechanism of action of the appliances is to rotate the mandible down and back, increasing the face height. The dental effects are to procline the upper incisors and retrocline the lower incisors.

Contra-indications

Due to the mechanism of action mentioned in the previous section, there are a number of circumstances in which a removable appliance should not be used to treat a reverse overjet. These are:

- Reverse overjet greater than 2 mm, without a mandibular displacement
- Skeletal discrepancy mainly in the mandible
- Lower anterior face height already increased
- Overbite reduced or frank anterior open bite

- Lower incisors already excessively retroclined
- Upper incisors already excessively proclined.

Types of appliance

The appliance types fall into two main categories: functional appliances and reverse headgear.

Functional appliances

Functional appliances are much more commonly used for the correction of Class II cases, as discussed above, but there are variations in the commonly used appliances for Class II cases that may be used to some effect in the treatment of Class III cases. These are the reverse Twin Block and the functional regulator III (FR III) appliances.

As with all functional appliances, the majority of the treatment effects are far more frequently on the dentition, rather than on the skeletal pattern. The treatment effects seen with the Class III functional appliances are:

- Retroclination of the lower incisors
- Proclination of the upper incisors
- Downward and backward rotation of the mandible, increasing the lower anterior face height
- Encouragement of forward growth of the maxilla.

This is why this treatment needs to be performed in a younger population than the Class II cases, as the maxilla stops growing considerably earlier than the mandible, often at least 2–3 years before the mandible stops growing.

Reverse Twin Block (Figures 10.12 and 10.13)

This appliance was also developed by Clark (1982). As with the Class II Twin Block, it consists of upper and lower blocks, and the following:

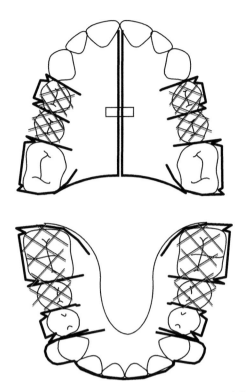

Figure 10.12 Diagrammatic representation of the design of a reverse Twin Block for correction of a reverse overjet associated with a mandibular displacement. Note the position of the acrylic blocks, which are positioned more anteriorly in the upper arch and more posteriorly in the lower arch, compared with a standard Twin Block (see Figure 10.3).

- Adams' clasps on upper and lower molars and first premolars
- Labial bow on the lower incisors
- Expansion screw as required
- Posterior acrylic blocks designed so that the lower one is held distal to the upper one.

Functional regulator III

A number of studies have shown the treatment benefits of this appliance, at least in the short term. It was developed by Rolf Fränkel and is also known as the Fränkel III appliance.

The FR III is a single appliance and is generally difficult for technicians to make (due to the complexity of the wire-work) and for operators to adjust. It is not clipped over the teeth, but relies on the patient's oral function to keep it in position, and so it may also be considered more difficult for the patient to tolerate than the reverse Twin Block.

The FR III consists of:

- Buccal shields to remove the constrictive effects of the buccinator muscle from the upper arch. These allow the upper arch to spontaneously increase in width.
- Acrylic labial pads in the upper labial sulcus to remove the effects of the obicularis oris muscle on the inclination of the upper incisors, allowing spontaneous proclination of the upper incisors.
- Labial bow on the lower incisors to cause retroclination of these teeth.

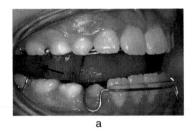
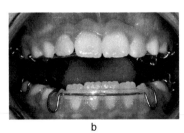
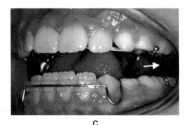

a   b   c

Figure 10.13 Intra-oral views of a reverse Twin Block *in situ*. Note the 45° slope of the upper (more anterior) and lower (more posterior) biteblocks (arrowed in a and c) as they interlock to provide a mesialising force on the maxillary dentition and a distalising force on the mandibular dentition. Compare this with the standard Twin Block shown in Figure 10.4. (Photographs courtesy of Andrew DiBiase.)

Reverse headgear

Reverse headgear is also known as a face-mask and may be used in conjunction with a URA or more commonly, with an expansion appliance bonded to the upper posterior teeth.

The reverse headgear is attached by elastic bands to hooks on the appliance in the primary molar region bilaterally. Anchorage for the forward movement of the maxilla is gained from pads that rest against the forehead and chin. The retention of a removable appliance needs to be excellent in order for the appliance not to be dislodged by the force of the elastic bands.

Many studies have indicated a short-term, positive treatment effect from reverse headgear attached to a bonded appliance. However, crucially, there are very few high-quality, prospective studies that are well-controlled and report on long-term follow-up of patients until the end of their growth period. See the article by Mandall *et al.* (2010) for a more detailed account of the use of this appliance.

All of the above appliances have been shown to work well in the short-term, depending on good patient cooperation. However, the fact that the mandible grows more and for longer than the maxilla means that the treatment outcome is liable to be unstable, and the use of these appliances for the definitive treatment of more severe Class III malocclusions in young children has yet to be proved conclusively.

References

Booth-Mason S, Birnie D (1988) Penetrating eye injury from orthodontic headgear–a case report. *European Journal of Orthodontics* **10**, 111–114

Clark WJ (1982) The Twin Block traction technique. *European Journal of Orthodontics* **4**, 129–138.

Clark WJ (1995) Twin Block Functional Therapy - Applications in Dentofacial Orthopaedics. Mosby, St Louis.

Mandall N, DiBiase A, Littlewood S, *et al.* (2010) Is early Class III protraction facemask treatment effective? A multicentre, randomized, controlled trial: 15-month follow-up. *Journal of Orthodontics* **37**, 149–161.

O'Brien K, Wright J, Conboy F, *et al.* (2003) Effectiveness of early orthodontic treatment with the Twin-block appliance: a multicenter, randomized, controlled trial. Part 1: Dental and skeletal effects. *American Journal of Orthodontics and Dentofacial Orthopedics* **124**, 234–243.

Vacuum-Formed Active Appliances

Jay Kindelan

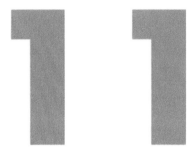

Orthodontic treatment is most commonly carried out using a combination of fixed and/ or removable appliances. From an orthodontist's perspective these appliances are capable of producing complex and accurate tooth movements. However, from a patient's perspective, they are usually unsightly and often uncomfortable to wear.

Several attempts have been made over the years at achieving orthodontic tooth movement with invisible appliances. Lingually placed fixed appliances do offer an aesthetic improvement; however, they provide significant compromise in terms of patient comfort and degree of difficulty for the orthodontic operator.

As long ago as 1945, Dr HD Kesling described the use of a flexible tooth-positioning appliance (Kesling, 1945). Within the last decade, several orthodontic companies have adapted vacuum-formed retainers (VFRs) to be used for the purpose of active orthodontic tooth movement (Tuncay, 2006). Different laboratory techniques are utilised in the construction of these

vacuum-formed active appliances (VFAAs). This chapter will focus on the clinical indications and potential limitations of such appliances.

Learning outcomes

At the end of this chapter you should be able to:

- Explain what VFAAs are
- Understand their limitations
- Understand some complications that can arise

Indications

It has been suggested that VFAAs are capable of achieving the vast majority of complex orthodontic tooth movements (Vlaskalic and Boyd, 2002; Boyd, 2008). However, it is our opinion that there are significant limitations to the tooth movement that can be achieved with VFAAs. VFAAs are particularly appropriate for simple tipping tooth movements; in addition,

Orthodontic Retainers and Removable Appliances: Principles of Design and Use, First Edition.
Friedy Luther and Zararna Nelson-Moon.
© 2013 Friedy Luther and Zararna Nelson-Moon. Published 2013 by Blackwell Publishing Ltd.

they are extremely effective at de-rotating teeth, even in cases that may prove troublesome with a fixed appliance. It has also been shown that prolonged orthodontic treatment with VFAAs may reduce anterior open bites due to the long-term intrusive forces produced by occlusal coverage of the posterior teeth.

Contra-indications

It is our opinion that VFAAs should not be used for complex orthodontic treatment, particularly involving dental extractions. VFAAs are not capable of producing bodily tooth movement. In addition it is extremely difficult to place intrusive or extrusive forces on individual teeth with VFAAs. Some authors have described the use of labial attachments placed on anchorage teeth to improve retention of the VFAA, allowing intrusive forces to be placed on adjacent teeth. However, the intrusion achieved is usually limited and often results in extrusion of the anchorage teeth.

Complications

Simple orthodontic problems can be treated with VFAAs within 6 months. However, prolonged use of VFAAs can lead to the development of mild posterior open bites due to the intrusive forces produced by full occlusal coverage of the appliances (Iscan and Sarisoy, 1997).

In view of the complete tooth coverage, oral hygiene and diet need to be excellent to prevent demineralisation, caries and periodontal problems.

General considerations

Types of cases

The majority of patients treated with VFAAs are adults who seek treatment complaining of incisor crowding. This can be related to a general dento-alveolar disproportion and is often exaggerated by poor tooth morphology.

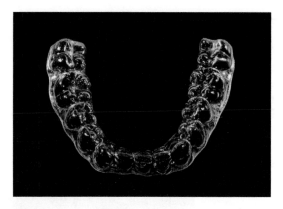

Figure 11.1 Aligner appliance corresponding to model eight in Figure 11.2.

Patients with crowded incisors often display relatively sharp contact points in addition to tapered crown form. The majority of adult cases treated with VFAAs require some interproximal reduction (IPR) during treatment. This provides space for alignment whilst flattening the contact points and is thought to enhance long-term stability. Systems that require mid-treatment impression taking do offer more flexibility when planning IPR. Often the required degree of IPR is difficult to specify at the start of treatment, and difficult to control precisely.

VFAA treatment is particularly suited to adult patients who are reluctant to consider fixed appliance treatment (Figure 11.1). In addition, there are advantages in adults who have heavily restored dentitions, with large numbers of crowns or veneers. Porcelain restorations have proved to be a challenge to orthodontic practitioners in terms of securing good attachment of fixed appliances. Obviously, this is not an issue when utilising VFAAs.

However, there are definite limitations of treatment with VFAAs and studies have shown that fixed appliances do produce consistently better results (Djeu *et al.*, 2005). It has been suggested that there may be less root resorption with VFAAs, but this area requires further research.

Manufacture

Most active tooth movement with VFAAs is planned around the most severely displaced tooth. Highly accurate silicone impressions are taken of the dental arch where tooth movement is planned. If no tooth movement is planned in the opposing arch, then an alginate impression will suffice to produce a standard orthodontic study cast to be used to determine the likeli-

hood of any occlusal interferences. Although some manufacturers do accept alginate impressions for production of working models, this may cause inaccuracies, particularly when impressions are posted to the laboratory.

The laboratory produces a series of aligning appliances, which gradually reduce the degree of displacement of the teeth to a point where alignment has been achieved (Figures 11.2 and 11.3). The degree of planned tooth movement

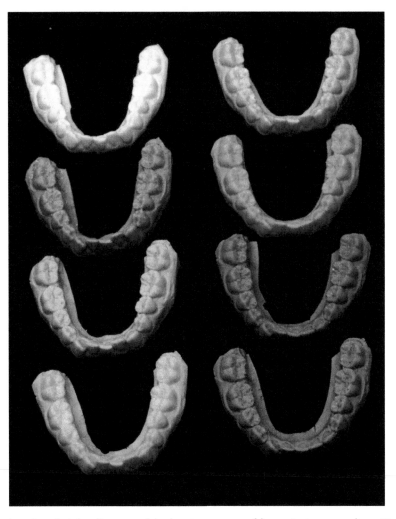

Figure 11.2   A series of eight aligner models showing a case of lower incisor crowding. Gradual improvement of the incisor position can be seen through the models. Completed alignment is not demonstrated by these models. (Reproduced with kind permission of Clearstep™.)

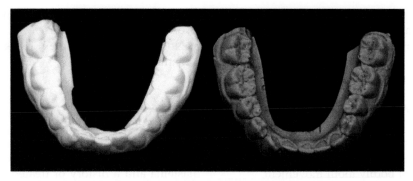

Figure 11.3 Working models used to produce stage one and stage eight aligners. This would demonstrate a time frame of 14 weeks between placement of aligner one and aligner eight. More treatment would be required to gain complete alignment. (Reproduced with kind permission of Clearstep™.)

between successive aligners varies between the different commercially available products. Tooth movement, however, is never planned to exceed 0.25 mm, which is generally accepted as the width of the periodontal ligament. In this way, orthodontic tooth movement is achieved by compressing the periodontal ligament on one side of the tooth root and creating tension on the opposite side, leading to bony remodelling.

The different commercial systems available vary in the provision of the aligning appliances. Most manufacturers plan treatment around a lead tooth, which is determined to move more than the other teeth during the alignment process. Some systems provide a series of eight aligners, which equate to 16 weeks of tooth movement. At that stage, a new set of silicone impressions is taken and a new series of aligning appliances constructed. Other manufacturers plan the entire treatment goals from the initial silicone impressions.

Some systems utilise computer plans to check and verify treatment goals prior to constructing aligner appliances. These computer goals can be extremely useful for patient information. A few authors suggest that inter-arch elastics can be used to apply Class II or Class III traction. In our opinion the application of inter-arch traction in this way is limited and in cases where significant sagittal correction is required, fixed appliances are indicated.

Wear of VFAAs

It is desirable that patients wear the appliances full time, apart from when eating, replacing the appliances once the teeth have been cleaned after meals. Less than full-time wear will result in delays in tooth movement and potential failure of treatment.

With most VFAA systems, an individual aligner will be worn for 2 weeks. When the aligner appliance is initially placed, it will feel tight on the patient's teeth but gradually, as the teeth move toward their initial pre-determined position, it will feel more comfortable on insertion and removal. After 2 weeks, the appliance can be easily inserted and removed, and the patient is instructed to move on to the next-stage aligning appliance.

At the completion of treatment some patients choose to wear their last aligner as a standard retention appliance. In other cases, bonded retainers are placed. Generally, bonded retainers will be placed in patients who have severe rotations before treatment or if it is considered that the teeth have been placed in an inherently unstable position (e.g. significant proclination of crowded lower incisors).

Some clinicians have expressed concerns about oral hygiene during treatment as the aligner appliances provide full dental coverage. However, it has been shown in several studies that plaque scores actually reduce during treatment, probably due to an increased dental awareness of the patients.

Summary

- Suitable for treatment of mild malocclusions
- Capable of tipping and de-rotating teeth
- Particularly suited to adult patients in view of good aesthetics
- Incapable of bodily tooth movement
- Severely limited use for intrusion and extrusion
- Long-term wear may cause posterior open bite

- May be helpful in treatment of mild anterior open bite
- Not ideal for complex cases involving extractions

Example cases

Case 1

An adult patient presented with a large midline diastema and a history of treated periodontal disease. On examination a maxillary midline diastema of 3.5 mm was present (Figure 11.4a and b). In addition, the patient had relative microdontia, which had been treated previ-

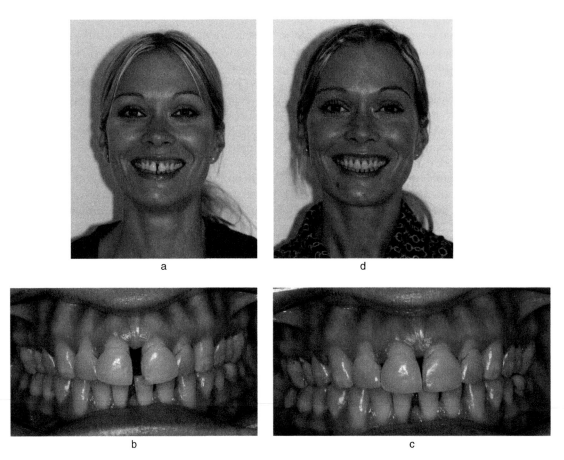

a

d

b

c

Figure 11.4 Case 1. (a) Patient smiling pre-treatment; (b) frontal view of teeth in occlusion pre-treatment; (c) frontal view of teeth in occlusion post-treatment; (d) extra-oral view post-treatment.

ously by placement of porcelain veneers on the four maxillary incisors. The patient was very keen to avoid placement of fixed appliances. Spacing was present in the lower incisor region but was of no concern to the patient.

Treatment was planned with VFAAs, tipping and approximating the four maxillary incisors with some palatal retraction. This was carried out over a 6-month period, utilising a series of 12 aligner appliances. At the end of treatment, the patient continued to wear her aligner appliance as a retainer (Figure 11.4c and d). This was subsequently replaced by a new VFR to provide a spare in case of loss or breakage. Placement of a bonded retainer on the palatal aspect of the incisors was considered; however, due to the relative microdontia, this would have led to

large spans of unsupported wire and likely fracture during normal wear. The patient continues to wear a VFR in bed at night long term.

Case 2

An adult patient presented with a severely rotated, crowded UR1 (Figure 11.5a and b). The tooth had previously suffered distal caries, causing difficulty with oral hygiene measures. The caries had been satisfactorily restored.

This adult patient expressed a disatisfaction with the prospect of wearing conventional fixed orthodontic appliances and therefore VFAAs were prescribed.

The teeth were aligned utilising a series of 16 aligners. At this interim stage, some interproximal

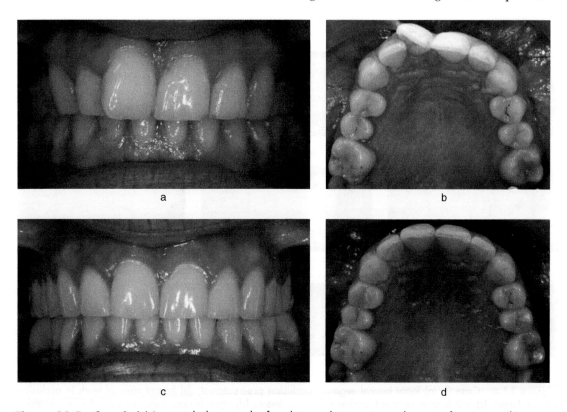

Figure 11.5 Case 2. (a) Intra-oral photograph of teeth in occlusion prior to the start of treatment; (b) mirror view of rotated maxillary right central incisor prior to start of treatment; (c) intra-oral photograph of teeth in occlusion after treatment; (d) mirror view of upper arch after treatment. (Reproduced with kind permission of Clearstep™.)

reduction was carried out and space closure subsequently completed with a further series of six aligners (Figure 11.5c and d). The patient continued to wear a VFR appliance at the end of active treatment on a nights-only basis long term. Placement of a bonded retainer was ill advised in this case due to the complete overbite present.

Case 3

An adult patient presented complaining of sticking out front tooth (proclined UR2; Figures 11.6a–c). They were unhappy about the prospect of wearing fixed appliances but were happy to wear VFAAs. The patient wore a

series of VFAAs (see progress in Figure 11.6d–f) and the finished result is shown in Figure 11.6g–j. The case shows the difficulty of intruding or levelling teeth; a fixed appliance would have been necessary to completely correct the UR2 position.

Case 4

An adult patient presented complaining of their twisted upper teeth tooth (the UR2 and UL2) and gap between their top front teeth. They too were unhappy about the prospect of wearing fixed appliances, but were happy to wear VFAAs. The pre- and post-treatment views are shown in Figure 11.7a–f.

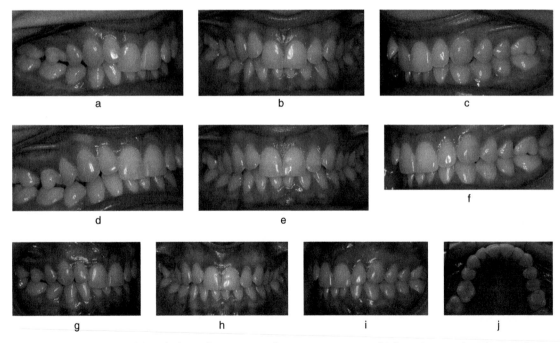

Figure 11.6 Case 3. (a) Right buccal segment occlusion pre-treatment; (b) frontal view of teeth in occlusion pre-treatment; (c) left buccal segment occlusion pre-treatment; (d) right buccal segment occlusion – treatment progress view; (e) frontal view of teeth in occlusion – treatment progress view; (f) left buccal segment occlusion – treatment progress view; (g) right buccal segment occlusion after treatment; (h) frontal view of teeth in occlusion after treatment; (i) left buccal segment occlusion after treatment; (j)mirror view of upper arch after treatment. Patient declined more aligners to complete, and was happy with outcome.

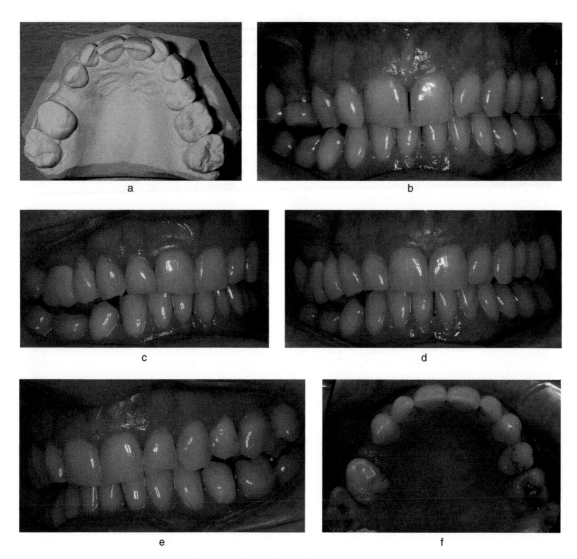

Figure 11.7 Case 4. (a) View of upper arch study model pre-treatment; (b) frontal view of teeth in occlusion pre-treatment; (c) right buccal segment occlusion post-treatment (with bridge); (d) frontal view of teeth in occlusion post-treatment; (e) left buccal segment occlusion post-treatment; (f) mirror view of upper arch after treatment.

References

Boyd RL (2008) Esthetic orthodontic treatment using the Invisalign appliance for moderate to complex malocclusions. *Journal of Dental Education* **72**, 948–967.

Djeu G, Shelton C, Maganzini A (2005) Outcome assessment of Invisalign and traditional orthodontic treatment compared with the American Board of Orthodontics Objective Grading System. *American Journal of Orthodontic Dento-Facial Orthoptics* **128**, 292–298.

Iscan HN, Sarisoy L (1997) Comparison of the effects of passive posterior bite-blocks with different construction bites on the craniofacial and dentoalveolar structures. *American Journal of Orthodontic Dento-Facial Orthoptics* **112**, 191–198.

Kesling HD (1945) The philosophy of the tooth-positioning appliance. *Journal of Dental Research* **31**, 297.

Tuncay OC (2006) *The Invisalign System*. Quintessence, London.

Vlaskalic V, Boyd RL (2002) Clinical evolution of the Invisalign appliance. *Journal of the Californian Dental Association* **30**, 769–776.

Index

Orthodontic Retainers and Removable Appliances: Principles of Design and Use, First Edition.
Friedy Luther and Zararna Nelson-Moon.
© 2013 Friedy Luther and Zararna Nelson-Moon. Published 2013 by Blackwell Publishing Ltd.

Printed and bound by CPI Group (UK) Ltd, Croydon, CR0 4YY

27/10/2024

14580388-0004